Music Therapy in Pediatric Healthcare: Research and Evidence-Based Practice

This publication was made possible through a grant
to the American Music Therapy Association
from The Recording Academy Grant Program,
a program of the
National Academy of Recording Arts & Sciences, Inc.

Music Therapy in Pediatric Healthcare: Research and Evidence-Based Practice

Edited by

Sheri L. Robb
University of Missouri–Kansas City

American Music Therapy Association, Inc.

Neither the American Music Therapy Association nor its Executive Board is responsible for the conclusions reached or the opinions expressed by the contributors to this book.

The American Music Therapy Association is a non-profit association dedicated to increasing access to quality music therapy services for individuals with disabilities or illnesses or for those who are interested in personal growth and wellness. AMTA provides extensive educational and research information about the music therapy profession. Referrals for qualified music therapists are also provided to consumers and parents. AMTA holds an annual conference every autumn and its eight regions hold conferences every spring.

For up-to-date information, please access the AMTA website at www.musictherapy.org

ISBN: 1-884914-10-1

The American Music Therapy Association, Inc.
8455 Colesville Road, Suite 1000
Silver Spring, MD 20910

Phone: (301) 589-3300
Fax: (301) 589-5175
Email: info@musictherapy.org
Website: www.musictherapy.org

Printed in The United States of America

Contents

Foreword

Music soothes the savage beast.
The beast that preys on children is probably the worst kind imaginable. Can music soothe beasts like sickle cell anemia, depression, premature births, AIDS, burns, seizures, birth defects, child abuse and cancer?

For children with these and other conditions, many days are filled with pain, tears and anxiety. Needle pokes, scans and visits to the operating room await many of them. There are medicines for them to take and doctors for them to see. It can be just as hard on the family as it is for the child. Doctors, nurses and other hospital personnel have to support the difficult times that these children and families have to endure. The toll on them is significant as well.

Professionals that work with children see on a daily basis that these are not little adults. Nor are they wild animals [well, okay, sometimes they are]. But these professionals get to see those fortunate times when they bounce back from the brink with few scars and fewer limitations. The message from these successes is that positive attitude is important. Although some kids with a positive attitude will die, without it, they rarely have a chance. Every child gets a prognosis, but they are human beings whose life is either zero or one hundred percent. This is not a game for them, nor is it fun. There is no point in trying for zero.

So what can music do?
It gives perspective. It connects. It redirects. It supports.
It remembers the past. It hopes for the future.
Music soothes.

When children are sedated for operations, music lets them know that they are not forgotten.
When babies lie in plastic incubators with their lives being supported by machines, music lets them know that there are parents waiting to hold them.
When adolescents are anxiously awaiting the next disappointment, music gives back some happier memories.

The effects quickly spread to families, friends and medical caregivers.
Parents do laundry and go back to work. Siblings go back to the business of playing. Doctors and nurses focus on medication schedules and comprehensive care.

All become soothed.

Soothe these savage beasts? Please read how music can try.
And enjoy.

The role of music therapy for children with medical needs is on-going at only a few academic locations. Its clinical efficacy, both emotionally and spiritually, is without question. The other answers regarding best practices and special areas of applicability will be forthcoming. Caregivers of children are encouraged to use music therapy to comfort, support, and connect with their patients.

Masayo Watanabe, M.D.
Pediatric Hematology/Oncology, The Children's Mercy Hospital
Assistant Professor of Pediatrics, University of Missouri–Kansas City

Introduction

Health care and helping professions have demonstrated a rapidly growing interest in evidence-based practice. The term *evidence-based practice* has been described as the adoption of interventions and practices that are informed by research (Dunst, Trivette, & Cutspec, 2002). Origins of the evidence-based approach to healthcare are traced to a British epidemiologist, Archie Cochrane, and his observations regarding the lack of ready access to reliable reviews of research to guide medical practice. In 1992, the Cochrane Collaboration was founded for the purpose of helping "...people make well informed decisions about health care by preparing, maintaining, and ensuring accessibility of systematic reviews of the effects of health care interventions" (Cochrane Collaboration, 2003, p. 3).

Music therapy is an established health care and human services profession that is dedicated to the implementation of controlled research studies to determine the underlying mechanisms in music that are responsible for therapeutic change, as well as clinical research to direct and guide the work of the music therapist. This growing body of research has enabled the music therapy profession to establish itself as a viable treatment modality for children in many areas, such as neurological rehabilitation and the use of music with premature infants. The power afforded by music therapy research, however, is limited if it is not readily accessible by the general public and medical community. Administrators and medical professionals often voice the need for hard evidence regarding the benefits of music therapy. This project, sponsored by the American Music Therapy Association (AMTA) and the National Association for Recording Arts & Sciences (NARAS), seeks to disseminate information on current research and evidence-based practices in pediatric music therapy to healthcare professionals and organizations across the United States.

In keeping with the philosophy of evidence-based practice, this publication begins with a meta-analysis of music therapy research with pediatric patients. This statistical procedure is used to examine a body of research for the purpose of identifying trends and generalizing results, and is used in medicine to justify clinical protocols. Subsequent chapters document the critical needs of specific patient populations and identify theories and research supporting the implementation of music-based interventions. This book highlights research and evidence-based practice methods that are being used in neonatal intensive care units, pediatric burn care, critical care and mechanical ventilation, neurological rehabilitation, chronic illness, procedural support, and surgical support.

You will notice that many of these chapters are written by music therapists in collaboration with other researchers and health care professionals. These collaborative relationships serve to strengthen our research and development of intervention protocols that are grounded in both basic science and clinical research. More importantly, collaborative work leads to better services for our patients and their families. I would like to dedicate this book to the more than 6 million children/adolescents and their families who experience hospitalization each year (Healthcare Cost and Utilization Project Website, 2001). They are an inspiration and keep us focused on identifying, developing, and providing the most efficacious treatment interventions possible. It is our hope that this publication, *Music Therapy in Pediatric Healthcare: Research and Evidence-Based Practice,* will provide the evidence necessary to increase availability of music therapy interventions in pediatric hospitals and units across the United States. We thank you for your interest in music therapy services for the patients and families that you serve each day.

Sheri L. Robb, PhD, MT-BC

References

Cochrane Collaboration. (1999). *Cochrane brochure.* Retrieved October 22, 2003 from http://www.cochrane.org/cochrane/cc-broch.htm

Dunst, C. J., Trivette, C. M., & Cutspec, P. A. (2002, September). Toward an operational definition of evidence-based practices. *Centerscope: Evidence-based approaches to early childhood development, 1*(1), 1 – 10. Retrieved from http://www.evidencebasedpractices.org/centerscope/centerscopevol1no.1pdf

Music therapy is an established health care and human services profession that uses music to improve quality of life by optimizing health and wellness. Highly trained and nationally certified music therapists build on the inherent qualities of music, using musical interventions in a focused and concentrated manner for healing and change, influencing physical, emotional, cognitive, and social responses. The National Association for Music Therapy, founded in 1950, and the American Association for Music Therapy, founded in 1971, came together in 1998 to form the American Music Therapy Association, ensuring the progressive development of the therapeutic use of music in education, medicine, and community settings. AMTA is the only professional music therapy organization in the United States, representing over 5,000 professionals.

ONE

∽

Music Therapy With Pediatric Patients: A Meta-Analysis

Jayne M. Standley, Ph.D., MT-BC
Jennifer Whipple, M.M., MT-BC

TRADITIONALLY, medical music therapy has thrived in settings with pediatric patients. Clinically, we have a great deal of literature and anecdotal evidence of effective practice. However, quantitative research and adequate documentation of these practices have accumulated slowly over the last 30 years. At this time, there is a moderately large body of quantitative research that merits review and assimilation.

Meta-analysis is a formal statistical procedure for synthesis of quantitative research data that provides more objective results than a traditional review of the literature. Its primary advantage is that more definitive conclusions about the efficacy of specific clinical procedures can then be derived (Mann, 1990). In the field of music therapy, meta-analysis originated with study of the efficacy of music in medical/dental treatment (Standley, 1986). That initial analysis found only 29 empirical studies. Over the years, this general medical/dental meta-analysis was updated twice (Standley, 1992, 1996) and found increasing bodies of research, 54 and 92 empirical studies, respectively. In the last update, only 19 studies with pediatric patients and 2 studies with NICU infants were identified.

In 2000, the trend in music therapy medical meta-analysis moved from global to specific with analyses of isolated medical procedures or patient groups in areas with an accumulation of at least 10 empirical studies. Effects have been analyzed for music therapy in surgery ($N = 13$ studies; Standley, 2000) showing music is far more effective when begun pre-operatively or post-operatively than during the surgery itself, and for MT with premature infants ($N = 10$ studies; Standley, 2002) showing music to be consistently effective across all Neonatal Intensive Care Unit applications. Additionally, Evans (2002) published a meta-analysis in a nursing journal on 19 studies using recorded music in medical treatment and concluded it to be effective for anxiety reduction.

Music therapy exclusively with pediatric patients has been included in only one meta-analysis. Kleiber and Harper (1999) reviewed the effects of distraction on children's pain and included three publications with music procedures. This analysis of 16 behavioral distress studies and 10 pain studies found mean effect sizes of .33 and .62, respectively, and concluded that distraction is an effective nursing intervention with hospitalized children. An earlier meta-analysis on pain intervention strategies with children showed no evidence of inclusion of music (Broome, Lillis, & Smith, 1989). Both of these analyses, however, revealed that pain responses of children are differentiated by age, with younger children having more severe reactions than children aged 4 years and above.

The purpose of this paper was to conduct a meta-analysis on empirical research studies contrasting music versus no music conditions during medical treatment of pediatric patients.

METHOD

Study Inclusion

Criteria for inclusion in this meta-analysis were:

1. Experimental studies using group or individual subject designs;
2. Studies with subjects who were pediatric patients between the age of term birth and 21 years who were receiving medical treatment in a medical setting, either a hospital, clinic, or doctor's office;
3. Studies with music utilized as a separate, independent variable contrasted with a no music control condition;
4. Studies with quantitative results reported with sufficient information to extract an effect size; and
5. Studies reported in the English language of design, procedures, and results amenable to replicated data analysis.

Pediatric studies with dental procedures, rehabilitation treatment in a non-hospital setting or omission of a control condition were excluded.

The procedures followed the four basic steps of a meta-analysis: (1) a complete literature search was conducted to find all possible members of the defined population of studies whether from published or unpublished sources; (2) the characteristics and qualities of the collected studies were identified, described, and coded; (3) these assigned codes were independently reviewed for reliability with discussion and re-review until full agreement was obtained, then (4) each study's results were statistically analyzed and converted to computed effect sizes using meta-analysis software (Johnson, 1989).

The identification process involved exhaustive searches of the *Journal of Music Therapy* (1964–present), *Music Therapy Perspectives* (1982–present), *Dissertation Abstracts* (1950–present), CINAHL (1982–present) and MEDLINE (1983–present). Keywords for searches of electronic indexes included children, child, pediatric, adolescent, neonate, and music. The reference lists of all identified articles and texts were also searched as were the bibliographies of two books in the field (Froehlich, 1996; Loewy, 1997).

Study Descriptions

Twenty-nine studies met criteria for inclusion in the meta-analysis. These studies are marked with an asterisk in the references and are summarized below.

- In the noninvasive procedural category, three studies investigated behavior state of term infants in the newborn nursery during background, recorded lullabies versus ambient noise (Kaminski & Hall, 1996; Lininger, 1987; Owens, 1979). There were also four pre-operative studies dealing with the child's anxiety that provided either live music therapy activities or music and relaxation procedures prior to surgery (Aldridge,1993; Chetta, 1980; Robb, Nichols, Rutan, Bishop, & Parker, 1995; Scheve, 2002). Several articles were unique. Ammon (1968) studied respiration rate of children under 2 years of age receiving high humidity respiration assistance during recorded music versus no music conditions. Froelich (1984) provided music therapy versus play therapy for children with a variety of illnesses on a pediatric unit. Grasso, Button, Allison, and Sawyer (2000) assessed enjoyment of children less than 2 years of age receiving chest physiotherapy treatment for cystic fibrosis during recorded versus no music conditions. Liebman and MacLaren (1991) studied anxiety of pregnant adolescents who received music and relaxation sessions prior to delivery. One study provided live music therapy sessions and assessed pre/post salivary IgA of children with a variety of diagnoses and severity levels (Lane, 1991).
- In the minor invasive procedures category, two studies looked at distress of newborn males during circumcision with recorded background music versus no music conditions (Joyce, Keck, & Gerkensmeyer, 2001; Marchette, Main, Redick, & Shapiro, 1989). Distress indicators of children receiving venipunctures for initiating IV lines were studied during recorded music (Arts et al., 1994) and during live music therapy sessions (Malone, 1996). Distress indicators were also measured during hypodermic injections with background music (Fowler-Kerry & Lander, 1987; Megel, Houser, & Gleaves, 1998). Self-report of pain was assessed by Lutz (1997) during laceration repair in the emergency room with recorded background music.
- In the major invasive procedures category, Clinton (1984) studied children receiving burn and cancer treatments during passive listening to background music. Schur (1986) and Pfaff, Smith, and Gowan (1989) investigated children receiving bone marrow aspirations while listening to background music. Schieffelin (1988) and Schneider (1982) assessed pain responses of children during wound debridement with live music therapy interactions. Siegel (1983) and Steinke (1991) conducted post-operative music and relaxation sessions for control of pain. Bradt (2001) evaluated a music entrainment procedure for post-operative pain. Two studies were conducted with children following their bone marrow aspirations and included live music therapy sessions, songwriting, and video production (Robb, 2000; Robb & Ebberts, in review).

We obtained and evaluated 26 additional pediatric music therapy articles which we determined to not meet our criteria for inclusion in the study. These included:

1. Studies without a no-music control condition (Barrera, Rykov, & Doyle, 2002; Caire & Erickson, 1986; Hanamoto & Kajiyama, 1974; Wade, 2002);
2. Studies not located in a medical setting (Behrens, 1982; Larson & Ayllon, 1990);
3. A study with parental data, but not pediatric data (Oggenfuss, 2001); and
4. A study with significant age difference between experimental and control groups which due to previous meta-analyses was considered a confounding variable (Gettel, 1985).

We also reviewed a number of articles and books with clinical descriptions of pediatric music therapy but no quantitative data (Bailey, 1984; Barrickman, 1989; Berlin, 1998; Brodsky, 1989; Cohen, 1984; Edwards, 1999; Fagen, 1982; Hoffman, 1975; Keller, 1995; Loewy, 1999; Marley, 1984; McDonnell, 1984; Micci, 1984; Rasco, 1992; Robb, 1996; Rudenberg & Royka, 1989; Slivka & Magill, 1986; Standley & Hanser, 1995).

Quality Analysis

Studies were coded for the following variables:

1. Published results: (a) medical source versus (b) music therapy source versus (c) unpublished source (theses/dissertations, papers presented at conferences, pre-publication papers);
2. Date of publication: (a) prior to 1990 versus (b) 1990 or later;
3. Type of medical procedure researched: (a) noninvasive procedures (patients hospitalized for general medical reasons, pre-surgery patients, newborns, etc. versus (b) minor invasive procedures such as venipuncture, hypodermic injections, and circumcision versus (c) major invasive treatment such as debridement, post-operative pain management, lumbar puncture, and post-bone marrow aspiration;
4. Subject age at time of study: (a) infant/toddler (term birth to < 4 years) versus (b) child (4 years to < 12 years) versus (c) adolescent (12 years or older) with coding determined by group mean.
5. Gender of subject pool: (a) more than 51% males versus (b) more than 51% females versus (c) equal number of each gender (49–51%);
6. Type of dependent variable: (a) physiologic (pulse, heart rate, respiration rate, salivary IgA, medication amount) versus (b) observed state (pain or distress indicators, crying) versus (c) emotional expressions (anxiety, depression);
7. Type of music: (a) session with live music versus (b) recorded music only;
8. Source of musical selection: (a) music therapist's professional judgment versus (b) patient preference (defined as all situations where the subject exercised any choice over musical content, either free choice or selection from menu of available music) versus (c) medical professional; and
9. Patient involvement with music: (a) active participation versus (b) passive listening.

Data Extraction

The value of one dependent variable from each study that contrasted music with a no-music control condition and that was considered the primary measurement of the study was converted to an estimated effect size, Cohen's *d* (Cohen, 1988). Table 1 shows the selected dependent variable and other qualities of each study that were coded for analysis. The earliest article was from 1968 and 55% of the studies were conducted by music therapists.

Table 1
Studies by Coded Qualities

Part A

Study Authors & Year	Publication Source	Medical Treatment Analyzed	Age	Gender
Aldridge (1993)	MT	Pre-Operative	Infant/Child[1]	Unknown[1]
Ammon (1968)	Medical	Humidified Respiratory Assistance	Infant	Mostly Females
Arts et al. (1994)	Medical	Venipuncture	Child	Mostly Males
Bradt (2001)	Unpublished MT Dissertation	Post-Operative	Adolescent	Mostly Males
Chetta (1980, 1981)[2]	MT	Pre-Operative	Child	Mostly Females
Clinton (1984)	Unpublished Medical Thesis	Painful Procedures for Cancer & Burn Patients	Child	Mostly Females
Fowler-Kerry & Lander (1987)	Medical	Hypodermic Immunization Injection	Child	Equal
Froelich (1984)	MT	General Pediatric Unit	Child	Mostly Males
Grasso et al. (2000)	Medical	Chest Physiotherapy for Cystic Fibrosis	Infant	Equal
Joyce et al. (2001)	Medical	Circumcision	Infant	Males
Kaminski & Hall (1996)	Medical	Newborn Nursery	Infant	Mostly Males
Lane (1991)	Unpublished MT Dissertation	General & Severe Diagnoses in Children's Hospital[1]	Child	Mostly Females
Liebman & MacLaren (1991)	MT	Pregnant Adolescents	Adolescent	Females
Lininger (1987)	Unpublished MT Thesis	Newborn Nursery	Infant	Mostly Females
Lutz (1997)	Unpublished Medical Thesis	Laceration Repair in ER	Child	Equal
Malone (1996; Batson, 1994)[2]	MT	Emergency Room & Pediatric Treatment Room Venipuncture	Infant	Mostly Males
Marchette et al. (1989)	MT	Circumcision	Infant	Males
Megel et al. (1998)	Medical	Hypodermic Immunization Injection	Child	Equal
Owens (1979)	MT	Newborn Nursery	Infant	Unknown
Pfaff et al. (1989)	Medical	Post Bone Marrow Aspiration	Child	Equal
Robb et al. (1995)	MT	Post-Operative	Child/ Adolescent[1]	Unknown
Robb (2000)	MT	Post-Bone Marrow Treatment	Child	Unknown

Study Authors & Year	Publication Source	Medical Treatment Analyzed	Age	Gender
Robb & Ebberts (in review)	Unpublished MT Paper	Pre, During, Post Bone Marrow Transplant	Adolescent	Mostly Females
Scheve (2002)	Unpublished MT Thesis	Pre-Operative	Child	Mostly Males
Schieffelin (1988)	Unpublished MT Conference Presentation	Debridement for Stevens-Johnson Syndrome	Infant	Male
Schneider (1982)	Unpublished Medical Dissertation	Burn Debridement	Adolescent	Mostly Males
Schur (1986)	Unpublished Medical Dissertation	Bone Marrow Aspiration & Lumbar Punctures	Ages 4–17[1]	Mostly Males
Siegel (1983)	Unpublished MT Thesis	Post Spinal Fusion Surgery	Unknown	Unknown
Steinke (1991)	MT	Post-Operative for Scoliosis	Adolescent	Equal

Table 1, Part B

Study	Type Dependent Variable	Independent Variables	Music Presentation	Music Selection	Music Interaction
Aldridge	Self-Report (Parental) of Child's Anxiety	MT Session vs. No Music	Live	Patient	Active
Ammon	Physiologic-Respiration Rate	Dvorak's *Symphony No. 5* vs. No Music	Recorded	Medical Professional	Passive
Arts et al.	Behavioral Observation of Pain Indicators	Contemporary, Upbeat Music vs. Placebo Emulsion Anesthetic	Recorded	Medical Professional	Passive
Bradt	Self-Report of Pain	Improvised Music for Entrainment vs. No Music	Live	Patient	Active
Chetta	Behavioral Observation of Distress Indicators	MT Sessions on Evening of Admission & Morning of Surgery vs. No Music	Live	MT	Active
Clinton	Self-Report of Pain	Music vs. No Music	Recorded	Patient	Passive
Fowler-Kerry & Lander	Self-Report of Pain	Music Suitable for Children vs. No Music	Recorded	Medical Professional	Passive
Froelich	Behavioral Observation of Anxiety Verbalizations	MT Sessions vs. Play Therapy	Live	MT	Active
Grasso et al.	Self-Report (Parental) of Child's Enjoyment	Physiotherapy with Music vs. No Music	Recorded	MT	Active

Study	Type Dependent Variable	Independent Variables	Music Presentation	Music Selection	Music Interaction
Joyce et al.	Behavioral Observation of Pain Indicators	Lullabies with Heartbeat vs. No Music	Recorded	Medical Professional	Passive
Kaminski & Hall	Behavioral Observation of High Arousal State	Classical Music vs. No Music	Recorded	Medical Professional	Passive
Lane	Physiologic – Salivary IgA	MT Sessions vs. No Music	Live	MT	Active
Liebman & MacLaren	Self-Report of Anxiety	Relaxation with Music vs. No Music	Recorded	MT	Active
Lininger	Behavioral Observation of Crying	Vocal Lullabies vs. No Music	Recorded	MT	Passive
Lutz	Self-Report of Pain	Music vs. No Music	Recorded	Patient	Passive
Malone	Behavioral Observation of Agitation/Crying	MT Session vs. No Music	Live	Patient	Active
Marchette et al.	Physiologic - Pulse Rate	Music vs. No Music	Recorded	Medical Professional	Passive
Megel	Behavioral Observation of Pain	Music vs. No Music	Recorded	Patient	Passive
Owens	Behavioral Observation of Crying	Lullabies vs. No Music	Recorded	MT	Passive
Pfaff et al.	Behavioral Observation of Distress Indicators	Music vs. No Music	Recorded	Patient	Active
Robb et al. (1995)	Self-Report of Anxiety	Music with Relaxation vs. No Music	Recorded	Patient	Active
Robb (2000)	Behavioral Observation of Pain Indicators	MT Sessions vs. No Music	Live	MT	Active
Robb & Ebbert (in review)	Self-Report of Depression	MT Sessions vs. No Music	Live	Patient	Active
Scheve	Self-Report of Anxiety	MT Sessions vs. No Music	Live	Patient	Active
Schieffelin	Behavioral Observation of Screams	MT Sessions vs. No Music	Live	Patient	Active
Schneider	Behavioral Observation of Pain Indicators	Music with Suggestion & Relaxation vs. No Music	Recorded	Patient	Active
Schur	Behavioral Observation of Distress Indicators	Music Listening vs. No Music	Recorded	Patient	Passive
Siegel	Physiologic – Amount of Pain Medication	Music with Relaxation vs. No Music	Recorded	MT	Active
Steinke	Physiologic - Amount of Pain Medication	MT Sessions vs. No Music	Recorded	MT	Active

[1] Variable could not be coded and was omitted from quality analysis.
[2] Some information was obtained from the unpublished thesis in addition to the publication resulting from the thesis.

Table 2
Results of Meta-Analysis

Study	*N*	*d*	95% CI	*r*	*p*
Aldridge	26	.84	+0.04 / +1.64	.41	.03
Ammon	20	2.61	+1.41 / +3.80	.81	.00
Arts et al.	120	–.05	- 0.41 / +0.31	–.03	.78
Bradt	32	1.51	+0.95 / +2.06	.61	.00
Chetta	50	.71	+0.14 / +1.28	.34	.02
Clinton	46	.20	-0.38 / +0.78	.10	.49
Fowler-Kerry & Lander	120	.39	+0.01 / +0.77	.19	.04
Froelich	39	.68	+0.04 / +1.33	.33	.04
Grasso et al.	20	1.06	+0.13 / +2.00	.49	.03
Joyce et al.	23	.87	+0.10 / +1.72	.41	.05
Kaminski & Hall	40	.76	+0.12 / +1.40	.37	.02
Lane	40	.13	-0.49 / +0.75	.07	.68
Liebman & MacLaren	39	2.02	+1.25 / +2.79	.72	.00
Lininger	24	.77	-0.05 / +1.60	.37	.07
Lutz	32	.73	+0.01 / +1.44	.35	.05
Malone	40	.14	-0.48 / +0.76	.07	.65
Marchette et al.	43	1.17	+0.51 / +1.82	.51	.00
Megel et al.	99	.47	+0.07 / +0.87	.23	.02
Owens	59	.05	-0.46 / +0.56	.03	.84
Pfaff et al.	12	.75	-0.42 / +1.92	.41	.17
Robb (1995)	20	.99	+0.06 / +1.92	.46	.04
Robb (2000)	20	1.35	+0.38 / +2.32	.59	.00
Robb & Ebberts (in review)	6	.65	-1.00 / +2.29	.37	.41
Scheve	60	.98	+0.44 / +1.51	.45	.00
Schieffelin	1	1.19	+0.57 / +1.80	.52	.00
Schneider	9	1.11	-0.30 / +2.53	.53	.12
Schur	26	.68	+0.12 / +1.24	.33	.01
Siegel	10	1.90	+0.31 / +3.49	.73	.01
Steinke	17	.21	-0.75 / +1.18	.11	.66
Overall:		.64	+0.52 / +0.76	.30	.00

N = 29 studies
Note. Q(28) = 76.131; *p* = .000
Total *N* = 1014 subjects. Mean *N*/study = 34.97

RESULTS

Table 2 lists each study, its sample size, the 95% confidence interval, the resulting Pearson *r* and Cohen's *d* statistics and their probability. Effect sizes ranged from –.05 to 2.61 with an overall mean effect size of .64 ($p = .00$). Since the 95% confidence interval did not include 0, this effect size is considered statistically significant and indicates that music therapy generally has a positive and significant impact in the medical treatment of children. The largest outlier was Arts, et al. (1994), a circumcision study with recorded background music that resulted in the only negative effect size. In this case, the effects of music were compared with those of a placebo analgesic cream. All other results were in a positive direction for the effects of music. The homogeneity Q-value was significant ($p = .00$) which means that the effect sizes of pediatric music therapy studies were inconsistent and not adequately explained by the single, mean effect size.

A quality analysis was conducted to identify reasons for inconsistency in the results. Results are shown in Table 3 with data by categories and subcategories. The homogeneity p indicates whether results by subcategory within a quality area were significantly different from each other. Six quality areas were significant and are marked with an asterisk. Essentially this table demonstrates that date of study did not differentiate results ($p = .64$) but publication source did ($p = .02$). The articles published in medical journals had significantly lower effect sizes.

With regard to subjects, age was significant ($p = .00$). Studies with adolescent subjects showed much greater benefit than did those with infants or children. Studies with infants had larger effect sizes than did those with children aged 4–12 years. Gender of subjects had no effect on results ($p = .28$).

The type of medical treatment did affect results ($p = .00$). Children with major invasive procedures (debridement, bone marrow aspirations, post-operative) and those with noninvasive procedures (pre-operative, chest physiotherapy, or newborn nursery) obtained significantly greater benefit from music therapy than did those having minor invasive procedures (venipunctures, circumcision, or hypodermic injections). These results may be due to flawed assumptions we made in operationally defining the subcategories. Or, perhaps the results reveal that the fear of a hypodermic injection, defined by us as a minor invasive procedure, is just as great for children as the fear of bone marrow aspirations or lumbar punctures defined as major invasive procedures.

With regard to type of dependent variable measured in the studies, those using behavioral observation had significantly lower effect sizes than did those using physiologic and self-report measures ($p = .02$).

Type of music was significant ($p = .03$) with live music resulting in greater benefit than recorded music. The person selecting the music did not cause differentiated study results. The music had similar effects whether selected by the music therapist, the patient, or the medical personnel. Music participation was significant ($p = .00$). Those actively involved with the music had significantly greater benefits than did those passively listening.

Figure 1 is a summary of clinical program guidelines and procedures for use of music with pediatric patients that were garnered from this research synthesis. Results of the meta-analysis strongly justify the incorporation of such music therapy techniques into the standard of care for children requiring medical services.

Table 3
Results of Quality Analysis

Quality Category	Homogeneity *p*	*N* Studies	*d*	95% CI	*r*	*p*
Date of Study						
Pre 1990	.64	13	.65	+0.47 / +0.83	.31	.01
1990–present		16	.63	+0.47 / +0.79	.30	.00
Publication Source	.02*					
Medical Journal		8	.43	+0.24 / +0.62	.21	.00
MT Journal		10	.71	+0.49 / +0.92	.33	.00
Unpublished		11	.82	+0.61 / +1.03	.38	.06
Dependent Variable						
Physiologic	.02*	5	.83	+0.45 / +1.21	.38	.00
Behavioral Observ.		14	.48	+0.32 / +0.64	.23	.04
Self-Report		10	.83	+0.63 / +1.03	.38	.00
Age of Subjects						
Infant < 4 years	.00*	9	.74	+0.51 / +0.97	.35	.00
Child 4–<12 years		11	.43	+0.27 / +0.59	.21	.07
Adolescent ≥12 years		5	1.36	+0.98 / +1.74	.56	.10
Gender of Subjects						
Mostly Males	.28	12	.68	+0.51 / +0.85	.32	.00
Mostly Females		7	.75	+0.48 / +1.03	.35	.00
Equal (49–51% ea.)		5	.47	+0.22 / +0.72	.23	.82
Medical Treatment						
Non-Invasive	.00*	10	.83	+0.62 / +1.05	.39	.00
Minor Invasive		7	.37	+0.19 / +0.56	.18	.05
Major Invasive		11	.91	+0.67 / +1.15	.41	.13
Music Type						
Live	.03*	10	.82	+0.61 / +1.03	.38	.05
Recorded		19	.55	+0.40 / +0.69	.26	.00
Music Selection						
MT	.14	10	.67	+0.44 / +0.90	.32	.00
Patient		13	.74	+0.56 / +0.92	.35	.11
Medical Professional		6	.46	+0.24 / +0.67	.22	.00
Music Participation						
Active	.00*	16	.89	+0.70 / +1.07	.40	.02
Passive		12	.44	+0.29 / +0.60	.22	.00

N = 29 studies
**p* < .05. Subcategories are not homogeneous and have significantly different results from each other.

OVERALL META-ANALYSIS RESULTS

- Music is significantly better than no music in pediatric medical treatment. All results were in a positive direction for benefits of music except one dependent variable in one study on circumcision of infants (overall $d = .64, p < .00$).
- Active music involvement is better than passive listening and live music is better than recorded.
- No differentiated effects by individual selecting music (patient vs. MT vs. medical personnel).
- MT functions better for noninvasive and major invasive procedures than for minor invasive procedures.
- Greatest effects are achieved for adolescents, then infants. Lesser effects occur for children aged 4–12 years.
- No differentiated effects by gender.
- Behavioral observation of pain and distress reveal modest effect sizes in comparison to physiologic and self-report measures of same.

MT CLINICAL OBJECTIVES FOR PEDIATRIC PATIENTS

I. Objectives Documented in the Quantitative Research Literature Included in the Meta-Analysis

A. Pain Reduction and Management for Invasive Procedures:

- surgical and post-operative treatments
- debridement
- bone marrow aspirations
- lumbar punctures
- venipunctures and hypodermic injections
- circumcision
- sutures

MT Techniques:

Live music activities with active participation and choices exercised by the patient
Music and relaxation techniques
Songwriting and video production about illness
Background, recorded music with passive listening (least effective)

B. Anxiety Reduction for

- pre-operative anxiety
- pre-treatment or repetitive, painful, invasive procedures
- pre labor and delivery

MT Techniques:
Live music activities with active participation and patient choice
Relaxation with music
Recorded music with instructions to focus on the music and/or suggestion

C. Infant Pacification
- newborn nursery

MT Techniques:
Recorded lullabies

D. Decreased Respiratory Distress
- children requiring respiratory assistance

MT Techniques:
Recorded background music with passive listening

E. Increased Coping Skills
- children receiving chest physiotherapy for cystic fibrosis
- children receiving bone marrow aspirations or lumbar punctures
- post-operative patients

MT Techniques:
Recorded music paired with physiotherapy
Music videos
Songwriting
Active participation in music activities

II. Objectives Cited in Other Literature

- nausea reduction
  hemodialysis
  chemotherapy
- mood elevation for depressed patients with serious illnesses
- reduction of developmental regressions through cognitive stimulation
  children with long-term hospitalization
  children with serious illnesses
- reinforcement and teaching of developmental milestones
- improved hospital-bound academic objectives
- increased socialization with peers, families, staff
- increased acceptance of, and coping skills, for illness/disability/disfigurement through counseling
- facilitation of expressions of discomfort or distress

- improved physical rehabilitation and development
  motor ability development through physical therapy exercises paired with music
  short-term memory enhancement
  stimulation for comatose patients
- improved speech and language rehabilitation
- increased respiratory capability through exercises paired with music or playing wind instruments
- improved neurologic development
  improved listening and auditory processing skills
  increased nervous system state regulation
- during radiology tests such as echocardiograms, CAT scans (eliminates need for sedation and RN supervision in almost all pediatric patients)
- provision of hospice MT for terminally ill children
- sleep inducement
- infant relaxation via therapeutic massage
- parent training/education

Figure 1. *Clinical Music Therapy Guidelines for Pediatric Patients*

CLINICAL IMPLICATIONS AND DISCUSSION

Meta-analysis of research with pediatric patients receiving medical treatments demonstrates that music therapy has a moderate to high effect, more so for adolescents than for other ages. This is consistent with other pediatric literature showing decreased benefits of pain interventions for younger children.

As with prior medical meta-analyses, the benefits of live music versus recorded background music were demonstrated (Standley, 2000). The presence of the music therapist allows for skillful intervention with ongoing adaptation to the emerging situation. This meta-analysis demonstrates that such involvement enhances benefits to the child.

In this meta-analysis, the mean sample size/study was 35. Though sample sizes in this area of research are small by medical standards, LeLorier, Gregoire, Benhaddad, Lapierre, and Derderian (1997) suggest that confidence in the validity of results is increased when certain conditions are met by a meta-analysis. These include the following, all characteristics of this study: overwhelming results in a positive direction with all studies except one showing greater benefits for music than for the control condition; clear *a priori* definitions for inclusion/exclusion of studies to reduce ambiguity of the collected body of literature; dual independent, objective analysis of studies to achieve concurrence in procedural decisions; and inclusion of published and unpublished work to avoid editorial bias.

Overall, this meta-analysis provides strong research evidence for many techniques and applications utilized in clinical music therapy. It also reveals critical gaps, since results of many procedures cited in the literature are not yet documented in empirical studies. Additional quantitative research is greatly needed with objectives beyond reduction of patient pain and anxiety.

As music therapists become more integrated into hospital treatment, we should strive for future research to meet the highest standards in the medical field: randomized clinical trials, large sample sizes of greater than 1,000 subjects, and controlled contrast of MT with alternative treatment interventions. Historically, music therapists have been active in developing pediatric research and have stimulated the medical field to follow suit. It would behoove us to continue to lead the quest for future documentation of our techniques.

REFERENCES

*Aldridge, K. (1993). The use of music to relieve pre-operational anxiety in children attending Day Surgery. *The Australian Journal of Music Therapy, 4*, 19–35.

*Ammon, K. J. (1968). The effects of music on children in respiratory distress. *American Nurses' Association Clinical Sessions*, 127–133.

*Arts, S. E., Abu-Saad, H. H., Champion, G. D., Crawford, M. R., Fisher, R. J., Juniper, K. H., & Ziegler, J. B. (1994). Age-related response to Lidocaine-Prilocaine (EMLA) emulsion and effect of music distraction on the pain of intravenous cannulation. *Pediatrics, 93*(5), 797–801.

Bailey, L. M. (1984). The use of songs in music therapy with cancer patients and their families. *Music Therapy, 4*(1), 5–17.

Barrera, M. E., Rykov, M. H., & Doyle, S. L. (2002). The effects of interactive music therapy on hospitalized children with cancer: A pilot study. *Psycho-Oncology, 11*, 379–388.

Barrickman, J. (1989). A developmental music therapy approach for preschool hospitalized children. *Music Therapy Perspectives*, *7*, 10–16.

*Batson, A. L. (1994). *The effects of live music on the distress of pediatric patients receiving intravenous starts, venipunctures, injections, and heel sticks*. Unpublished master's thesis, The Florida State University, Tallahassee.

Behrens, G. A. (1982). *The use of music activities to improve the capacity, inhalation, and exhalation capabilities of handicapped children's respiration*. Unpublished master's thesis, Kent State University, Kent, OH.

Berlin, B. K. (1998). Music therapy with children during invasive procedures: Our emergency department's experience. *Journal of Emergency Nursing, 24*(6), 607–608.

*Bradt, J. (2001). *The effects of music entrainment on postoperative pain perception in pediatric patients*. Unpublished doctoral dissertation, Temple University, Philadelphia, PA.

Brodsky, W. (1989). Music therapy as an intervention for children with cancer in isolation rooms. *Music Therapy, 8*(1), 17–34.

Broome, M. E., Lillis, P. P., & Smith, M. C. (1989). Pain interventions with children: A meta-analysis of research. *Nursing Research, 38*(3), 154–158.

Caire, J. B., & Erickson, S. (1986). Reducing distress in pediatrics patients undergoing cardiac catheterization. *Children's Health* Care, *14*(3), 146–152.

*Chetta, H. D. (1980). *The effect of music therapy in reducing fear and anxiety in preoperative pediatric patients.* Unpublished master's thesis, The Florida State University, Tallahassee.

*Chetta, H. D. (1981). The effect of music and desensitization on pre-operative anxiety in children. *Journal of Music Therapy, 18*(2), 74–87.

*Clinton, P. K. (1984). *Music as a nursing intervention for children during painful procedures.* Unpublished master's thesis, The University of Iowa, Iowa City.

Cohen, J. (1988). *Statistical power analysis for the behavioral sciences* (2nd ed.). Hillsdale, NJ: Lawrence Erlbaum Associates.

Cohen, Z. N. (1984). *The development and implementation of a pediatric music therapy program in a short-term medical facility.* Unpublished master's thesis, New York University, New York.

Edwards, J. (1999). Anxiety management in pediatric music therapy. In C. Dileo (Ed.), *Music therapy and medicine: Theoretical and clinical applications* (pp. 69–76). Silver Spring, MD: American Music Therapy Association.

Evans, D. (2002). The effectiveness of music as an intervention for hospital patients: A systematic review. *Journal of Advanced Nursing, 37*(1), 8–18.

Fagen, T. S. (1982). *Music therapy as a tool for the assessment and treatment of fear and anxiety in pediatric cancer patients.* Unpublished master's thesis, New York University, New York.

*Fowler-Kerry, S., & Lander, J. R. (1987). Management of injection pain in children. *Pain, 30,* 169–175.

*Froehlich, M. R. (1984). A comparison of the effect of music therapy and medical play therapy on the verbalization behavior of pediatric patients. *Journal of Music Therapy, 21*(1), 2–15.

Froehlich, M. R. (Ed.). (1996). *Music therapy with hospitalized children.* Cherry Hill, NJ: Jeffery Books.

Gettel, M. K. (1985). *The effect of music on anxiety in children undergoing cardiac catheterization.* Unpublished master's thesis, Hahneman University, Philadelphia, PA.

*Grasso, M. C., Button, B. M., Allison, D. J., & Sawyer, S. M. (2000). Benefits of music therapy as an adjunct to chest physiotherapy in infants and toddlers with cystic fibrosis. *Pediatric Pulmonology, 29,* 371–381.

Hanamoto, J., & Kajiyama, T. (1974). Some experiences in use of environmental music in pediatric roentgenography. *Radiologia Diagnostica, 15*(6), 787–794.

Hoffman, P. (1975). The use of guitar and singing in a child life program. *Journal of the Association for the Care of Children in Hospitals, 4*(1), 45–47.

Johnson, B. T. (1989). DSTAT: Software for the meta-analytic review of research literature. Hillsdale, NJ: Lawrence Earlbaum Associates.

*Joyce, B. A., Keck, J. F., & Gerkensmeyer, J. (2001). Evaluation of pain management interventions for neonatal circumcision pain. *Journal of Pediatric Healthcare, 15*(3), 105–114.

*Kaminski, J., & Hall, W. (1996). The effect of soothing music on neonatal behavioral states in the hospital newborn nursery. *Neonatal Network, 15*(1), 45–54.

Keller, V. E. (1995). Management of nausea and vomiting in children. *Journal of Pediatric Nursing, 10*(5), 280–286.

Kleiber, C., & Harper, D. (1999). Effects of distraction on children's pain and distress during medical procedures: A meta-analysis. *Nursing Research, 48*(1), 44–49.

*Lane, D. L. (1991). *The effect of a single music therapy session on hospitalized children as measured by salivary Immunoglobulin A, speech pause time, and a patient opinion Likert scale*. Unpublished doctoral dissertation, Case Western Reserve University, Cleveland, OH. (UMI No. 9137062)

Larson, K., & Ayllon, T. (1990). The effects of contingent music and differential reinforcement on infantile colic. *Behavior Research and Therapy, 28*(2), 119–125.

LeLorier, J., Gregoire, G., Benhaddad, A., Lapierre, J, & Deriderian, F. (1997). Discrepancies between meta-analyses and subsequent large randomized, controlled trials. *The New England Journal of Medicine, 337*(8), 536–542.

*Liebman, S. S., & MacLaren, A. (1991). The effects of music and relaxation on third trimester anxiety in adolescent pregnancy. *Journal of Music Therapy, 28*(2), 89–100.

*Lininger, L. W. (1987). *The effects of instrumental and vocal lullabies on the crying behavior of newborn infants*. Unpublished master's thesis, Southern Methodist University, Dallas, TX.

Loewy, J. V. (Ed.). (1997). *Music therapy and pediatric pain.* Cherry Hill, NJ: Jeffrey Books.

Loewy, J. V. (1999). The use of music psychotherapy in the treatment of pediatric pain. In C. Dileo (Ed.), *Music therapy and medicine: Theoretical and clinical applications* (pp. 189–206). Silver Spring, MD: American Music Therapy Association.

*Lutz, W. G. (1997). *The effect of music distraction on children's pain, fear, and behavior during laceration repairs*. Unpublished master's thesis, The University of Texas at Arlington.

*Malone, A. B. (1996). The effects of live music on the distress of pediatric patients receiving intravenous starts, venipunctures, injections, and heel sticks. *Journal of Music Therapy, 33*(1), 19–33.

Mann, C. (1990). Meta-analysis in the breech. *Science, 249,* 476–480.

*Marchette, L., Main, R., Redick, E., & Shapiro, A. (1989). Pain reduction during neonatal circumcision. In R. Spintge & R. Droh (Eds.), *MusicMedicine* (pp. 131–136). Ann Arbor, MI: Malloy Lithographing.

Marley, L. S. (1984). The use of music with hospitalized infants and toddlers: A descriptive study. *Journal of Music Therapy, 21*(3), 126–132.

McDonnell, L. (1984). Music therapy with trauma patients and their families on a pediatric service. *Music Therapy, 4*(1), 55–63.

*Megel, M. E., Houser, C. W., & Gleaves, L. S. (1998). Children's responses to immunizations: Lullabies as a distraction. *Issues in Comprehensive Pediatric Nursing, 21*(3), 129–145.

Micci, N. O. (1984). The use of music therapy with pediatric patients undergoing cardiac catheterization. *The Arts in Psychotherapy, 11*, 261–266.

Oggenfuss, J. W. (2001). *Pediatric surgery and patient anxiety: Can music therapy effectively reduce stress and anxiety levels while waiting to go to surgery?* Unpublished master's thesis, The Florida State University, Tallahassee.

*Owens, L. D. (1979). The effects of music on the weight loss, crying, and physical movement of newborns. *Journal of Music Therapy, 16*(2), 83–90.

*Pfaff, V., Smith, K., & Gowan, D. (1989). The effects of music-assisted relaxation on the distress of pediatric cancer patients undergoing bone marrow aspirations. *Children's Health Care, 18*(4), 232–236.

Rasco, C. (1992). Using music therapy as distraction during lumbar punctures. *Journal of Pediatric Oncology Nursing, 9*(1), 33–34.

Robb, S. L. (1996). Techniques in song writing: Restoring emotional and physical well being in adolescents who have been traumatically injured. *Music Therapy Perspectives, 14*(1), 30–37.

*Robb, S. L. (2000). The effect of therapeutic music interventions on the behavior of hospitalized children in isolation: Developing a contextual support model of music therapy. *Journal of Music Therapy, 37*(2), 118–146.

*Robb, S. L., & Ebberts, A. G. (in review). Songwriting and digital video production interventions for pediatric patients undergoing bone marrow transplantation part I: An analysis of depression and anxiety levels according to phase of treatment.

*Robb, S. L., Nichols, R. J., Rutan, R. L., Bishop, B. L., & Parker, J. C. (1995). The effects of music assisted relaxation on preoperative anxiety. *Journal of Music Therapy, 32*(1), 2–21.

Rudenberg, M. T., & Royka, A. M. (1989). Promoting psychosocial adjustment in pediatric burn patients through music therapy and child life therapy. *Music Therapy Perspectives, 7*, 40–43.

*Scheve, A. M. (2002). *The effect of music therapy intervention on pre-operative anxiety of pediatric patients as measured by self-report.* Unpublished thesis, The Florida State University, Tallahassee.

*Schieffelin, C. (1988, April). *A case study: Stevens-Johnson Syndrome*. Paper presented at the Annual Conference, Southeastern Conference of the National Association for Music Therapy, Tallahassee, FL.

*Schneider, F.A. (1982). *Assessment and evaluation of audio-analgesic effects on the pain experience of acutely burned children during dressing changes*. Unpublished doctoral dissertation, University of Cincinnati, Cincinnati, OH. (UMI No. 8228808)

*Schur, J. M. (1986). *Alleviating behavioral distress with music or Lamaze pant-blow breathing in children undergoing bone marrow aspirations and lumbar punctures.* Unpublished doctoral dissertation. The University of Texas Health Science Center at Dallas, Dallas, TX.

*Siegel, S. L. (1983). *The use of music as treatment in pain perception with post-surgical patients in a pediatric setting*. Unpublished master's thesis, The University of Miami, Coral Gables, FL.

Slivka, H. H., & Magill, L. (1986). The conjoint use of social work and music therapy in working with children of cancer patients, *Music Therapy, 6A*(1), 30–40.

Standley, J. M. (1986). Music research in medical/dental treatment: Meta-analysis and clinical applications. *Journal of Music Therapy, 23*(2), 56–122.

Standley, J. M. (1992). Meta-analysis of research in music and medical treatment: Effect size as a basis for comparison across multiple dependent and independent variables. In R. Spintge & R. Droh (Eds.), *MusicMedicine* (pp. 364–378). St. Louis: MMB.

Standley, J. M. (1996). Music research in medical/dental treatment: An update of a prior meta-analysis. In C. Furman (Ed.), *Effectiveness of music therapy procedures: Documentation of research and clinical practice* (2nd ed., pp.1–60). Silver Spring, MD: National Association for Music Therapy.

Standley, J. M. (2000). Music research in medical treatment. In AMTA (Ed.), *Effectiveness of music therapy procedures: Documentation of research and clinical practice* (3rd ed., pp. 1–64). Silver Spring, MD: American Music Therapy Association.

Standley, J. M. (2002). A meta-analysis of the efficacy of music therapy for premature infants. *Journal of Pediatric Nursing, 17*(2), 107–113.

Standley, J. M., & Hanser, S. B. (1995). Music therapy research and applications in pediatric oncology treatment. *Journal of Pediatric Oncology Nursing, 12*(1), 3–8.

*Steinke, W. R. (1991). The use of music, relaxation, and imagery in the management of postsurgical pain for scoliosis. In C. Maranto (Ed.), *Applications of music in medicine* (pp. 141–162). Washington, DC: National Association for Music Therapy.

Wade, L. M. (2002). A comparison of the effects of vocal exercises/singing versus music-assisted relaxation on peak expiratory flow rates of children with asthma. *Music Therapy Perspectives, 20*(1), 31–37.

*Studies included in this meta-analysis.

Two

Music Therapy for Premature Infants in the Neonatal Intensive Care Unit: Health and Developmental Benefits

Jayne M. Standley, Ph.D., MT-BC
Jennifer Whipple, M.M., MT-BC

DEVELOPMENTAL NEEDS IN THE NICU

MEDICAL SCIENCE has made amazing progress in understanding the neurological development of the fetus and subsequent abilities of the newborn infant. It is apparent that infant learning typically begins in the womb. In the third trimester the human fetus is adding an astounding number of brain cells, over 200,000 per minute. Normally, these cells begin immediately to migrate, racing to link up with a specific neurological function. Learning begins with these migrations and is dependent upon genetic endowment interacting with environmental opportunity for intellect and abilities to develop. Gestational weeks 24–40 are a fertile and critical learning period for the fetus. Any interruption of this process by drugs, alcohol, disease, or premature birth is detrimental to long-term well-being.

Unfortunately, the incidence of premature births in America is increasing, as is survivability. Infants born as early as 24 weeks gestational age have a 50% chance of living while those born only a few weeks later have an 80–90% chance of survival. The premature infant remains in the Neonatal Intensive Care Unit (NICU) until approximately his/her original due date. This means that the youngest babies spend the entire third trimester of fetal development unbuffered by the womb.

At the time of greatest neurological development, premature infants live in a hospital NICU, not a womb or a quiet home setting. Their post birth experiences include painful and stressful medical procedures highly correlated with increased long-term impairment in neurological development. Physical and environmental constraints limit learning opportunities as do treatments and nourishment scheduled according to medical priorities, not infants' indications of desire for food or attention.

Additionally, many aspects of the NICU environment are extremely aversive to the developmentally immature infant. These include around the clock lighting without night/day cycles, alarms at attention-getting decibel levels, and mechanical noises of ventilator-assisted breathing and incubator heat pumps. Such an environment produces high and persistent stress that forestalls normal brain cell migration and can ultimately "wire" the brain in a hyper-alert state. In addition to stress factors, some life sustaining medical treatments damage developing sensory abilities: high volumes of oxygen to assist breathing can cause permanent visual impairment while some life-saving drugs are ototoxic and damage hearing ability for life.

The neurological implications of premature birth are particularly problematic with a high risk for lifelong impairment, need for special education, and notably reduced brain volume apparent up to 8 years later (Peterson et al., 2000). Premature infants are likely to require special education services for hyperactivity, learning disabilities, cerebral palsy, or mental retardation. Many will have increased medical costs throughout the developing years. Since the brain continues maturation throughout life, it is fortunate that some neurological problems can be mitigated by nurturing and carefully structured developmental learning opportunities beginning as early as possible. Medical treatment options for the severely premature child are far more advanced than developmental interventions, but mounting concern about long-term outcomes is placing cautious emphasis on identifying safe, effective early intervention in the NICU.

The medical community places primary emphasis on eliminating as many stimuli as possible from the stress-producing NICU environment to assure maximum opportunity for infant sleep and rest that promotes neurological development. The addition of music therapists' contact with their accompanying auditory stimuli is sometimes viewed with concern by NICU staff. However, it is known that complex environments are better for learning than simple, deprived ones. Research also shows with normally developing infants that the earlier intervention begins the better. Critical and sensitive periods of brain development require that particular stimuli must be available during windows of opportunity for maturation in that particular area (Greenough, Emde, Gunnar, Massinga, & Shonkoff, 2001). Music is a noninvasive, nurturing stimulus that can be therapeutically used to accomplish developmental and medical objectives throughout the infant's stay in the NICU and is an important stimulus for the development of aural perception skills.

RATIONALE FOR MT IN THE NICU

The NICU environment is filled with auditory stimuli, most of which are undesirable. It is imperative that the music therapist provide an explanation for the differences between musical sounds and ambient noise and provide a solid rationale for their insertion into the NICU.

A critical developmental fact is that hearing begins to develop early in gestation and all infants need continuing nonstressful aural stimulation to acquire auditory perception skills. As early as 16–18 weeks gestation, fetal heart rate begins to respond to loud sounds denoting that hearing is emerging. By 28 weeks this response to auditory stimuli is consistent. From this point to 38–40 weeks full-term development, the fetus is hearing maternal sounds and responding to them. Fetuses in the womb during the third trimester begin to discriminate among speech sounds, particularly with regard to pitch and rhythm. At birth, term newborns can recognize their mother's voice, pick out a particular story read during the last month of fetal development, and discriminate components of their native language, including awareness of grammar, syntax, and specific language phonemes. Auditory exposure from birth, whether term or premature, is absolutely critical to the further development and specification of auditory abilities, including the most critical skill of language development.

Preterm infants reside in an atypical environment largely deficient in the sounds which start the language learning process. Especially critical is the fact that the human voice frequencies can be masked by those of the ventilator, incubator or other ambient noises in the NICU. Therefore, premature infants can spend long periods of time missing critical auditory processing opportunities and many show long-term developmental deficits as a result. Carefully chosen sung music can, to a limited extent, compensate for this loss of important auditory input.

Music has unique acoustic properties that make it a positive masking agent for ambient noise. Ambient sounds are incidental, not chosen or present for therapeutic reasons. They exist in the environment without controls for volume, duration, location, or desirable cause/effect relationships. The inconsistent characteristics of noise, irregular frequencies and inconsistencies of tension, stress and configuration, produce fatigue and stress in the listener, especially a premature infant with an immature neurological system. Intentional sounds such as music are chosen for their potential to soothe and provide exposure to complex auditory stimuli that promote appropriate neurological stimulation.

Aural perception requires the translation of sound vibrations and normally begins developing during the last trimester in utero. Music is a distinctive auditory stimulus with many cognitive elements neurologically processed both simultaneously and in sequence. The neurological system concurrently perceives melody, rhythm, harmony, timbre, form, style, and expressive characteristics as it also retains, orders this information across time, and contrives aural expectancies. Acoustically, then, music is unique sound. It is more pleasant, soothing, and interesting than noise and uses highly preferred frequencies and harmonics selected through centuries of refinement and development of the music system. One rationale for music in the NICU is that listening to music promotes neurological organization.

Music used in the NICU must soothe infants while masking ambient sound. Lullabies are a preferred choice for music therapy since they can promote language development while facilitating the infants' sleep and rest cycles. It is known that language development is faster if vocal stimuli are individually directed to the infant, as in live singing. Language development is also faster when stimuli include extended vowels, mellifluous sounds, narrow pitch ranges rising for stimulation and falling for pacification, and repeated pitch contours (Trehub, Unyk, & Trainor, 1993). These characteristics are present in the lullabies of all cultures. Using lullabies from the family's culture can also contribute to normalizing the preterm infant's third trimester of development. So, sung lullabies can stimulate language development, soothe the infant, and individualize the environment with culturally relevant selections.

GUIDELINES FOR MUSIC SELECTION

The following guidelines were developed from the research literature for the selection of recorded and live music appropriate for the NICU and for the design of clinical music therapy and research protocols:

- Recorded or live music in the NICU should be soothing, constant, stable, (i.e., relatively unchanging since changing auditory stimuli are alerting). Nonalerting music contains these elements: voice *a cappella* or with only one accompanying instrument, stable rhythm with light emphasis, constant volume, and melodies in the higher vocal ranges which infants hear best. Major modes are less disquieting than minor modes. Music therapists can consult with parents and make efforts to obtain or record appropriate arrangements of their preferred music. The same selection should be used repetitively for greatest pacification especially when the infant is very young and most fragile. A variety of calming selections can be used later for developing auditory processing skills.
- The human voice, especially that of the mother, promotes bonding while also exposing the infant to language. Since very premature infants have not had the opportunity to hear the mother's voice daily in the womb, they need opportunities to learn to recognize her. When the mother or music therapist is present, individually-directed, culturally appropriate live music is much preferred to recorded music. Research shows that singing is more effective than speaking for soothing the infant.
- Music should be presented individually and binaurally. Volume should not exceed 65–70 dB (Scale C) measured at the infant's ear. Care must be taken to set the loudness level individually to meet the readiness level for each baby, the logistics of his/her care environment, and to assure that nearby infants are not disturbed. For this reason, unit-wide, free field music is not recommended.
- Music therapy can generally begin for infants around 28 gestational weeks if medical status permits. Infants as young as 24 gestational weeks have shown no ill effects from music presentation, though research is scarce in this age range. These very young children may be considered candidates if medical status permits and the parents agree.
- Music duration should not exceed a total of 1.5 hours/day alternating in 30-minute segments. Very young infants or those displaying reduced oxygen saturation levels at music cessation should receive shorter periods of stimulation (4–5 minutes) fading in and out and alternating with equal periods of silence. The nurse providing daily care for the infant should verify that he/she could benefit from sound stimulation before music is initiated. Many times the infant has endured medical procedures, is ill, is demonstrating symptoms of overstimulation, or is generally in need of the greatest amount of rest possible. The nurse is the best authority to decide if it is appropriate to play recordings or to determine that music should be terminated at any time.
- Musical toys and mobiles are almost always contraindicated. They provide sounds or melodies of short duration that are repetitive, often their volume cannot be controlled, and their sound cannot be localized. They can add to ambient noise in other infants' environment and frequently the sound quality is poor.
- There is as yet no long-term research on the effects of extended music stimulation on hearing capability and ongoing development of the inner ear. Music therapists should be aware of the fragility of this process and err on the side of caution in terms of length and type of music presentation.

GUIDELINES FOR NICU TRAINING

Prior to working in the NICU, Music therapists should review confidentiality and liability issues as defined by the risk management division of the hospital in which they will provide services and should also acquire professional practice liability insurance. Then, they should acquire full knowledge of the clinical setting by completing specialized training. Such training entails understanding the following:

- NICU protocols for clinical services, roles of interdisciplinary team members in assessment and treatment planning, and involvement and rights of parents in treatment decisions;
- Professional confidentiality regarding infants and families, particularly with regard to life-sustaining treatment or its cessation, paternity issues, cultural and socioeconomic factors, very young mothers making decisions for their infants, and diverse lifestyles;
- Nonjudgmental acceptance of infants' status and parent/staff decisions regarding treatment or its withholding;
- Health and infection control issues, including the importance of staff not coming to the nursery when exhibiting symptoms such as: cold, runny nose, diarrhea, fever, fever blister, exposure to chicken pox; the avoidance of artificial nails which can house and spread bacteria; and the use of universal precautions in the presence of bodily fluids (gloves and avoidance of needles and disposal bins);
- Scrubbing and glove requirements for diapering or stimulating infants as indicated by the medical staff;
- Discrimination of permissive interactions such as diapering, holding and rocking infants, and offering a pacifier versus nonpermissive interactions such as feeding;
- The necessity for daily approval from the primary caregiver to provide music therapy for an individual infant;
- Music therapy techniques for premature infants;
- Recognition of warning signs of infant distress and protocols for discontinuation of interaction;
- Knowledge of medical conditions and treatments affecting premature infants' ability to participate in music therapy interventions.

NICU RESEARCH AND DOCUMENTED MT CLINICAL TECHNIQUES

A decade of music research with premature infants in the NICU has resulted in 10 studies published in nursing or music therapy journals or presented at major conferences. A recent meta-analysis of this research demonstrated highly significant effects of almost a standard deviation due to music treatment (overall effect size $d = .8268$, $p < .001$) (Standley, 2002). Results were homogeneous indicating consistent, highly positive benefits across all studies. That is, diverse applications of music provided significant positive effects for premature infants across a variety of physiological and behavioral variables: observed behavior state, heart rate, respiration rate, oxygen saturation level, weight gain, days in hospital, feeding rate, and nonnutritive sucking rate. Table 1 contains a list of the studies and their dependent variables included in the meta-analysis.

Table 1
Characteristics of NICU Music Studies Included in Meta-Analysis

Study	Independent Variables Tested in Experimental/ Control Conditions	Adjusted Gestational Age of Infants	Dependent Variable Showing Significant Results
Caine (1991)	Lullabies vs. ambient noise	Unknown	Days in hospital Weight gain Behavior state
Cassidy & Standley (1998)	Lullabies vs. ambient noise	27 wks.	Oxygen saturation
Coleman et al. (1997)	Lullabies vs. ambient noise	29.5 wks.	Heart rate Oxygen saturation Behavior state Days in hospital Weight gain
Collins & Kuck (1996)	Lullabies with heart beats vs. ambient noise	30 wks.	Oxygen saturation Behavior state Heart rate
Flowers (1999)	'70s Ballads and lullabies with heart beats vs. ambient noise	28 wks.	Oxygen saturation Behavior state
Moore, Gladstone, & Standley (1997)	Lullabies vs. white noise	31 wks.	Oxygen saturation
Standley (1998)	Live singing of lullabies with multimodal stimulation vs. ambient noise	30.6 wks.	Days in hospital Weight gain
Standley (2000a)	Recorded lullabies contingent upon pacifier suck vs. ambient noise	35.5 wks	Nonnutritive sucking rate
Standley (2003)	Recorded lullabies contingent upon pacifier suck vs. ambient noise	36.1 wks.	Feeding rate
Standley & Moore (1995)	Recorded lullabies vs. ambient noise	Unknown	Oxygen saturation

Music therapy is a profession with a rich history of benefits to developmental intervention. Music activities can be utilized to promote a wide array of cognitive growth, social interaction, and motor coordination skills in early childhood and have been a traditional component of curricula for infant stimulation and early childhood education (Davis, 2001). These same techniques are important for the older infant who may remain hospitalized for many additional months or even life long care.

However, music therapy for the fragile newborn NICU infant must be carefully selected and documented as medically safe and beneficial. For each procedure recommended in this chapter, the research in the area was reviewed and "best practice" clinical procedures synthesized. It has been reported that well-intentioned, but unresearched provision of music in the NICU has included harpists, earth drums to simulate the sound of the mother's heart, classical music recordings to promote intelligence since the misleading media assumptions about "Mozart makes you smart," and piped in, unit-wide music including that from radio stations. The effects of these practices are as yet undocumented. Therefore, their usage is questionable at this time and not included here.

Research has identified three primary uses of NICU music therapy that promote growth and development in the premature infant. These are the bases for clinical music therapy in the NICU and include:

1. Music to mask aversive environmental stimuli and reduce stress thereby promoting physiological well-being and stability;
2. Music to assist neurological maturation and teach tolerance to stimulation; and
3. Music to reinforce nonnutritive sucking.

Music to Stabilize Behavior State, Oxygen Saturation, and Respiration Rate

Length of hospitalization is reduced by almost a week when recorded lullabies are played for approximately 1.5 hours per day throughout the premature infant's NICU stay (Caine, 1991). With NICU services costing thousands of dollars per day for each infant, this is potentially an important health care savings. However, the greatest benefit may come from removing the children from the NICU and placing them into a home environment with family care and bonding, day/night cycles of light and darkness, and social interactions that promote learning.

Research shows that infants maintain homeostasis during music listening (Standley, 1998). To accomplish this the music must be as unchanging as possible with consistent tempo and volume, simple melody and simple instrumentation and accompaniment. Such music combined with the human voice in the form of a lullaby pacifies and has the added bonus of conveying language concepts.

It should be noted that recorded music must be provided at appropriate volume levels to protect the still developing inner ear. With regard to noise, the American Academy of Pediatrics recommends that ambient levels not exceed 55 dB (Scale A) in the NICU 24-hour environment (American Academy of Pediatrics, 1997). Music (measured on Scale C) has been played at a variety of dB levels (Cassidy & Ditty, 1998). Current consensus is that 65 dB (Scale C) measured at the infant's ear is most effective (which approximates 55 dB measured on Scale A). It should be placed binaurally to stimulate both ears equally and is faded in and out to reduce the possibility of startling the infant.

The infant's behavior state consists of five phases on a continuum from crying through active alert, quiet alert, and quiet sleep to the deepest sleep. Brain wave analysis shows that growth and neurological development occur during periods of active (REM) sleep through which the infant cycles for up to 20 minutes at a time (Gardner, Garland, Merenstein, & Lubchenco, 1997).

Caregivers try to not interrupt periods of active (REM) sleep by scheduling all interventions in one period followed by a period of reduced stimuli to enhance the chance of the infant sleeping. Music listening can be scheduled immediately following painful procedures to help the infant transition from a distressed to a sleep state and to maintain homeostasis. After a short term of up to 30 minutes, it is faded out and the infant is allowed to rest undisturbed. If physiological monitors indicate greater fluctuations without music than with music, then music can be faded in again. The music may be faded in and out for ½ hour intervals for no more than 1.5 hours total listening time.

In addition to homeostasis, premature infants listening to music demonstrate increased oxygen saturation and stable respiration rates (Cassidy & Standley, 1995; Coleman, Pratt, Stoddard, & Gerstmann; Collins & Kuck, 1991; Flowers, McCain, & Hilker, 1999; Moore, Gladstone, & Standley, 1994; Standley & Moore, 1995). During rises in saturation levels, the amount of oxygen may be reduced by the respiratory therapist. Lesser amounts of oxygen decrease potential harm to the infant's developing vision. Greater stability of physiological responses also reduces instances of apnea and bradycardia.

Music for Tolerance to Stimulation

Music and touch have been shown to enhance neurological development (Gardner et al., 1997; Standley, 1998). Additionally, stroking promotes breathing in the neonate when the neurological system is mature enough to tolerate it (Gardner et al., 1997). Therefore, massage and touch are excellent therapies for premature infants beginning at approximately 30 weeks gestation. Due to an immature neurological system, the premature infant is hypersensitive to stimuli and all stimuli are cumulative. The younger the infant's gestational age, the more easily he/she is overwhelmed by stimuli and all stimuli must cease if an infant becomes hyperresponsive. Faster habituation to changing stimulation without hyperresponsivity equates to greater neurological maturation.

The multimodal stimulation procedure was developed initially with the speaking voice used as the stimulus to contact the infant (Burns, Cunningham, White-Traut, Silvestri, & Nelson, 1994). A procedure combining quiet humming and progressive tactile stimulation has shown that music maintains homeostasis and promotes tolerance for increasing levels of multimodal stimulation (Standley, 1998).

In this procedure, the infant is held without movement or stroking while a lullaby is hummed slowly, monotonously, and quietly. If the infant remains pacified, then slow, firm stroking begins. This touch uses moderate pressure and slow, rhythmic repetitions. Stroking progresses in the same manner that the neurological system matures (i.e., cephalocaudally and proximodistally, from the head down and the center of the body outward). If these stimuli are tolerated, then vestibular (slow rocking) and visual stimuli (eye-to-eye contact) are attempted sequentially. All cuddling and/or social responses are reinforced with differentiated soothing verbalizations using the infant's name.

If any signs of overstimulation are noted at any point in the above procedure, then all stimulation ceases. These signs are myriad and include yawning, hiccoughing, or sneezing; tongue protrusion; finger splay or outstretched arm; struggling movements; averted or clinched eyes; flushed, blotchy, or pale skin color; grimacing or creasing forehead into a frown; startle reflex response in which infants extend their necks and throw out their arms and legs; hyperalertness as evidenced by a wide-eyed, fixed stare; whimpering, crying, or cry face; spitting or vomiting; irregular heart rate or respiratory rate; oxygen saturation level dropping below 86%; and limp body or lack of responsiveness. Research has shown that this procedure results in greater average weight gain per day and significantly shorter hospitalization for female infants (Standley, 1998). It can be used therapeutically as soon as 31.5 weeks adjusted gestational age (Whipple, 2002).

Also within the framework of music and multimodal stimulation is parent training in the procedure. Medical staff often chastise parents to avoid overstimulating the fragile infant with whom they eagerly wish to interact. However, parents are seldom trained in appropriate interactive techniques. Results of a study examining effects of parent training in multimodal stimulation indicated significantly fewer infant stress behaviors, more appropriate parent interaction with, and responses to infants, and more time spent in hospital visitation for parents who received instruction in appropriate uses of music and multimodal stimulation techniques (Whipple, 2000).

Parents of premature infants often experience stress due to infant prognosis and treatment, the financial burden of their infant's initial hospitalization and future care, and the necessity of learning to become responsible for life-saving care procedures. The implementation of parent training in music and multimodal stimulation can provide parents a positive method of interaction with their hospitalized infant, facilitating bonding and optimal development even in this stressful environment. In addition, parents can transfer the interaction skills to caregiving procedures and extend the music and multimodal stimulation benefits beyond hospitalization.

Music for Increasing Nonnutritive Sucking

The NICU environment is designed to deliver medical care. Subsequently, care is provided according to medical priorities, not infant reactions to the environment. Since learning at the beginning of life is based on reciprocal environmental cause/effect relationships, the premature infant needs early intervention opportunities to engage in such relationships. Music has been shown to be an effective reinforcer for teaching new behaviors to term infants in the first year of life (Standley, 2001) and to increase nonnutritive sucking rates (Standley, 2000).

The infant's sucking ability is a critical behavior for both survival and neurological development. Sucking is the first rhythmic behavior in which the developing infant engages and its appearance is highly correlated with the appearance of brain wave activity in the fetus (Goff, 1986). Therefore, nonnutritive sucking is theorized to contribute to neurological development by facilitating internally regulated rhythms. It also increases infant pacification and oxygenation. Time spent in nonnutritive sucking is a natural behavior of third trimester fetuses in the womb, but medical and environmental constraints often inhibit sucking opportunities in the NICU. Some infants must later be taught this skill.

A pacifier fitted with a pressure transducer and timer allows short segments of music to be contingent upon nonnutritive sucking (Standley, 2000). Research has shown that premature infants learn to control the music duration within about 2.5 minutes and more than double their sucking rates during the first learning opportunity with such a mechanism. Astonishingly, premature infants learn as quickly as older infants under conditions of music reinforcement (Standley & Madsen, 1990). Surprisingly, the ability to learn this basic cause/effect skill is not dependent upon further maturation.

Research has shown that premature infants can benefit from increased nonnutritive sucking skill during feeding training (Standley, 2003). At 34 weeks gestation, premature infants are ready to move from gavage to nipple feeding. The suck-swallow-breathe coordination necessary for nipple feeding must sometimes be taught after the premature infant has been tube fed for an extended period. Often physical therapy is attempted to facilitate sustained feeding attention, capability, and sucking responses strong enough to allow infants to gain adequate daily nutrition by mouth. This training is expensive and time consuming, and often fails. Music reinforcement for nonnutritive pacifier sucking has resulted in improved feeding rates (Standley, 2003). It is theorized that use of the mechanism results in the infant's producing sucking bursts followed by pauses to listen to music. At the next nipple feeding opportunity, this seems to improve the requisite pacing skill necessary for extended periods of sucking to accomplish feeding.

CONCLUSION

Research-based music therapy improves the quality of life for premature infants. It also promotes specific, immediate neurological benefits during the medical and developmental crisis of a NICU stay. Music can mask aversive stimuli, pacify in the presence of changing stimuli, stabilize vital functions, and reinforce active behavior change. It promotes these positive changes without detrimental side effects, a novel attribute in the problematic neonatal intensive care environment.

Research in this area is too new to determine whether other, longer term developmental consequences also accrue. However, results are conclusive enough to justify cautious clinical applications of very early early intervention with music.

REFERENCES

American Academy of Pediatrics. Committee on Environmental Health. (1997). Noise: A hazard for the fetus and newborn. *Pediatrics, 100*(4), 724–727.

Burns, K., Cunningham, N., White-Traut, R., Silvestri, J., and Nelson, M. (1994). Infant stimulation: Modification of an intervention based on physiologic and behavioral cues. *Journal of Obstetric, Gynecologic, and Neonatal Nursing, 23*(7), 581–589.

Caine, J. (1991). The effects of music on the selected stress behaviors, weight, caloric and formula intake, and length of hospital stay of premature and low birth weight neonates in a newborn intensive care unit. *Journal of Music Therapy, 28*(4), 180–192.

Cassidy, J. W., & Ditty, K. M. (1998). Presentation of aural stimuli to newborns and premature infants: An audiological perspective. *Journal of Music Therapy, 35*(2), 70–87.

Cassidy, J. W., & Standley, J. M. (1995). The effect of music listening on physiological responses of premature infants in the NICU. *Journal of Music Therapy, 32*(4), 208–227.

Coleman, J. M., Pratt, R. R., Stoddard, R. A., Gerstmann, D. R., & Abel, H.-H. (1997). The effects of the male and female singing and speaking voices on selected physiological and behavioral measures of premature infants in the intensive care unit. *International Journal of Arts Medicine, 5*(2), 4–11.

Collins, S. K., & Kuck, K. (1991). Music therapy in the Neonatal Intensive Care Unit. *Neonatal*

Network, 9(6), 23–26.

Davis, R. K. (2001). Taking first steps in preschool together: A hierarchical approach to group music therapy intervention. *Early Childhood Connections, 7*(2), 33–43.

Flowers, A. L., McCain, A. P., & Hilker, K. A. (1999). *The effects of music listening on premature infants.* Paper presented at the Biennial Meeting, Society for Research in Child Development, April 15–18, Albuquerque, NM.

Gardner, S., Garland, K., Merenstein, S., & Lubchenco, L. (1997). The neonate and the environment: Impact on development. In G. B. Merenstein & S. L. Gardner (Eds.), *Handbook of neonatal intensive care* (4th ed., pp. 564–608). St. Louis: Mosby.

Goff, D. M. (1986). The effects of nonnutritive sucking on state regulation in preterm infants. *Dissertation Abstracts International, 46,* 8B, 2835.

Greenough, W., Emde, R., Gunnar, M., Massinga, R., & Shonkoff, J. (2001). The impact of the caregiving environment on young children's development: Different ways of knowing. *Zero to Three, 21*(5), 16–23.

Moore, R., Gladstone, I., & Standley, J. (1994). *Effects of music, maternal voice, intrauterine sounds and white noise on the oxygen saturation levels of premature infants.* Unpublished paper presented at the National Conference, National Association for Music Therapy, November, Orlando, FL.

Peterson, B. S., Vohr, B, Staib, L. H., Cannistraci, C. J., Dolberg, A., Schneider, K. C., Katz, K. H., Westerveld, M., Sparrow, S., Anderson, A. W., Duncan, C. C., Makuch, R. W., Gore, J. C., & Ment, L. R. (2000). Regional brain volume abnormalities and long-term cognitive outcome in preterm infants. *Journal of the American Medical Association, 284*(15), 1939–1947.

Standley, J. M. (1998). The effect of music and multimodal stimulation on physiologic and developmental responses of premature infants in neonatal intensive care. *Pediatric Nursing, 24*(6), 532–538.

Standley, J. M. (2000). The effect of contingent music to increase nonnutritive sucking of premature infants. *Pediatric Nursing, 26*(5), 493–499.

Standley, J. M. (2001, Spring). The power of contingent music for infant learning. *Bulletin of the Council for Research in Music Education, 149,* 65–71.

Standley, J.M. (2002). A meta-analysis of the efficacy of music therapy for premature infants. *Journal of Pediatric Nursing, 17*(2), 107–113.

Standley, J. M. (2003). The effect of music-reinforced nonnutritive sucking on feeding rate of premature infants. *Journal of Pediatric Nursing, 18*(3), 169–173.

Standley, J. M., & Madsen, C. K. (1990). Comparison of infant preferences and responses to auditory stimuli: Music, mother, and other female voice. *Journal of Music Therapy, 27*(2), 54–97.

Standley, J. M., & Moore, R. (1995). Therapeutic effects of music and mother's voice on premature infants. *Pediatric Nursing, 21*(6), 509–512, 574.

Trehub, S. E., Unyk, A., & Trainor, L. (1993). Adults identify infant-directed music across cultures. *Infant Behavior and Development, 16*(2), 193–211.

Whipple, J. (2000). The effect of parent training in music and multimodal stimulation on parent-neonate interactions in the Neonatal Intensive Care Unit. *Journal of Music Therapy, 37*(4),

250–268.

Whipple, J. (2002, April). Implications of early referral for music and multimodal stimulation in the Neonatal Intensive Care Unit: A pilot study. Paper presented at the annual conference of the Southeastern Region of the American Music Therapy Association, Macon, GA.

THREE

Music Therapy in Pediatric Burn Care

Christine Tuden Neugebauer, M.S., MT-BC
Volker Neugebauer, M.D., Ph.D.

THE USE OF MUSIC THERAPY as a treatment modality for burn patients is a growing field. The pioneering work of Christenberry (1979) was the first to describe the practice of music therapy in the burn population. Not until 10 years later did clinicians further explore its application to pediatric burn patients (Rudenberg & Royka, 1989). Since then, research developments in the music therapy profession have evolved and now include both qualitative and quantitative analyses for both adult and pediatric burn populations. Nevertheless, music therapy research with this specialized group still remains in its early stages.

In order to develop and validate effective protocols for treating pediatric burn patients using music therapy, clinicians must extrapolate research findings from other disciplines. Music as treatment tool is tremendously flexible by nature and can be integrated systematically with other therapeutic approaches. Cross-disciplinary research findings from the fields of pain, traumatology, psychology, rehabilitation science, and medicine highlight the direction of treatment options that music therapy offers to pediatric burn care.

HISTORICAL PERSPECTIVE

Serious interest in exploring the application of music therapy in pediatric medicine started about two decades ago. However it was not until the end of that first decade when Rudenberg and Royka (1989) provided the first comprehensive overview of music therapy in pediatric burn care. This article addressed many important psychosocial and physiological concerns in burn recovery. In particular, the review focused on how both music therapy and child life interventions could be implemented during treatment. In the 1990s more summative articles began to appear in the music therapy literature. These articles provided a clinical framework and rationale for using music with burn-injured children (Daveson, 1999; Edwards, 1994, 1998). An increasing number of case studies were also published during this time. These case narratives covered pertinent topics related to burn care such as coping during wound debridement and facilitating emotional adjustment (Edwards, 1995; Loveszy, 1991). In addition, Bishop, Christenberry, Robb, and

Rudenberg (1996) elaborated on the primary issues involved in pediatric burns and illustrated psychosocial treatment processes using detailed case descriptions.

An experimental study, Robb, Nichols, Rutan, Bishop, and Parker (1995) reported that music-assisted relaxation alleviated preoperative anxiety in pediatric burn patients undergoing plastic and reconstructive surgery. More recently, Fratianne et al. (2001) discovered that two specific interventions, music-based imagery and musical alternate engagement, significantly decreased self-reported pain perception during debridement as compared to the control group.

Because music therapy is primarily a clinical and patient oriented profession with a relatively small research base, it is critical for music therapists to synthesize research findings from other disciplines. Pediatric burn injuries are devastating and often require long-term physical and emotional recuperation. To be effective the music therapist must possess the versatile skills necessary to treat the many complex psychosocial, physiological, and rehabilitative needs of the burn-injured child.

PATHOPHYSIOLOGY OF BURN INJURY

Skin, the largest organ in the human body, has many fascinating roles. Regulating body temperature, preventing loss of body fluids, protecting the body from harmful microorganisms, physical and chemical factors, and providing a variety of sensations, including touch and pain, are all important functions necessary for human survival. When a substantial portion of skin becomes injured, grave adverse reactions occur throughout the body. Treatment for a severe burn injury involves fluid resuscitation, metabolic support, respiratory care, body temperature control, protection against infection, and wound management (Herndon, 2002; Tarnowski, 1994). Depending upon the severity of the injury, patients may undergo numerous operative procedures for excision and skin grafting. Length of hospitalization varies with the severity of burn(s) and can range from a few days to several months. A severe burn injury can be devastating: it may necessitate the amputation of digits or extremities and result in orthopedic complications as well as moderate to severe physical disfigurement.

Types of burns include scald, flame, chemical, electrical, and contact injuries. Injuries may result from house fires, occupational hazards, motor vehicle accidents, self-immolation, negligence or even child abuse. Children are considered a high-risk population for sustaining burn injuries with an estimated 83,000 children receiving emergency treatment in 1997 alone (Herndon, 2002). Scientific advances in the medical management of burn injuries have resulted in the significant increase of survival rate from massive burns. More and more children are living after sustaining burns that cover more than 50% of their total body surface area (TBSA). Once the child has surpassed the acute stage of injury, the overall recovery process will continue with ongoing plastic and reconstructive surgical procedures (Herndon, 2002). These children require intensive psychological and social support from the moment of injury through rehabilitation to facilitate their adjustment to this devastating and potentially life-changing injury.

PAIN

In burn care, pain is an inevitable part of the healing process and presents one of the greatest challenges for clinicians working on the burn unit. However, prior to discussing the treatment applications of music therapy, it is important to understand the underlying mechanisms and different components involved in the pain experience.

Pain Mechanisms

> Pain is a critical national health problem. It is the most common reason for medical appointments, nearly 40 million visits annually, and costs this country over $100 billion each year in health care and lost productivity. Pain has a profound effect on the quality of human life. In addition to possible deleterious effects on immune function, pain can cause disruptions in sleep, eating, mobility, and overall functional status. In the hospitalized patient, pain may be associated with increased length of stay, longer recovery time, and poorer patient outcomes, all of which have health care quality and cost implications.
> (*NIH* Guide, Biobehavioral Pain Research, PA-03-152, 2003)

Pain evoked by a transient stimulus that is not associated with significant tissue damage serves as a physiological warning for a potentially tissue-damaging situation. A "noxious" stimulus is detected by specialized endings of nerve fibers in the peripheral tissue (skin, muscles, joints, viscera) and converted into electrical signals, which are transmitted to nerve cells (neurons) in the spinal cord. Spinal cord neurons activated by noxious stimuli send nociceptive signals along their axons in several "pain pathways" to various brain areas, including thalamus, cortex and limbic system.

Different from transient nociception are prolonged and chronic pain states, which arise from pathological lesions such as injury and inflammation. A key factor in prolonged and chronic pain is neural plasticity—the capacity of neurons in the peripheral and central nervous system to change their function, chemical profile, or structure. Enhanced excitability of peripheral nerve fibers and of neurons in the central nervous system (CNS) is referred to as peripheral and central sensitization, respectively. Sensitization is both the consequence and a key mechanism of persistent pain states; it is associated with phenomena like hyperalgesia, i.e., increased pain sensitivity, and allodynia, i.e., pain due to a normally nonpainful stimulus (Basbaum, 1999; Dubner & Gold, 1999; Fields & Basbaum, 1999; Neugebauer, 2002; Stucky, Gold, & Zhang, 2001; Willis, 2002; Wood & Perl, 1999; Woolf & Salter, 2000; Yaksh, Hua, Kalcheva, Nozaki-Taguchi, & Marsala, 1999).

Despite significant progress in pain research over the past two decades and the discovery of a variety of chemicals in the peripheral and central nervous system ("transmitters") that act to regulate the formation and transmission of "pain signals" along the pain neuraxis, persistent pain remains difficult to treat and has a profound effect on the quality of human life. "Pain is personal and subjective, is affected by mood and psychosocial factors, and demonstrates tremendous individual variation" (*NIH* Guide, Management of Chronic Pain, PA-01-115, 2001). Hope for new therapeutic strategies lies in a better understanding of pain mechanisms and factors that influence pain experience as well as in the study and inclusion of approaches outside the standard treatments such as pain medication.

Different Components of Pain

Pain is a multi-dimensional experience that includes sensory-discriminative (i.e., localization and intensity), cognitive-conscious (reasoning, catastrophizing, personalization) and emotional-affective (anger, fear, anxiety, depression) components. The sensation of pain is highly dynamic (Heinricher & McGaraughty, 1999; Rhudy & Meagher, 2000). Emotional responses and affective states and disturbances are associated with persistent pain conditions and can modify the experience of pain (Heinricher & McGaraughty, 1999; Rhudy & Meagher, 2000). In fact, a reciprocal relationship exists between pain and negative affect (Huyser & Parker, 1999; Ohayon & Schatzberg, 2003): persistent pain results in anxiety and depression (Huyser & Parker, 1999) and patients suffering from anxiety and depression experience pain more strongly (Haythornthwaite, Sieber, & Kerns, 1991). Thus, for novel and improved therapeutic strategies it is crucial to consider the whole spectrum of pain and related phenomena and to "explore basic mechanisms of the conscious perception of pain and the affective responses to pain" (*NIH* Guide, Biobehavioral Pain Research, PA-03-152, 2003).

Accumulating evidence points to the amygdala as a neural substrate of the reciprocal relationship between pain and emotion (McGaraughty & Heinricher, 2002; Meagher, Arnau, & Rhudy, 2001). The amygdala complex is a medial temporal lobe brain structure, which is generally believed to be involved in the neural substrates of emotion. As part of the limbic system the amygdala plays a key role in the emotional–affective aspects of behavior, the emotional evaluation of sensory stimuli, emotional learning and memory, reinforcement and motivation, but also related disorders such as anxiety and depression (Aggleton, 2000).

Importantly, intensely pleasurable responses to music correlate with decreased activity in the amygdala (Blood & Zatorre, 2001). It has been suggested that music may maximize pleasure through inhibition of brain areas associated with negative emotions such as the amygdala (Blood & Zatorre, 2001). In fact, such action may be an important mechanism by which music therapy exerts its beneficial effects on pain experience and tolerance.

It has become clear now that the amygdala is also part of the pain system and is well positioned to play a key role in the emotional–affective component of pain. Neuroimaging pain studies using positron emission tomography (PET) and functional magnetic resonance imaging (fMRI) have repeatedly identified pain-related signal changes in the amygdala in animals and humans (Becerra et al., 1999; Bingel et al., 2002; Bonaz et al., 2002; Bornhovd et al., 2002; Derbyshire et al., 1997; Paulson, Casey, & Morrow, 2002; Schneider et al., 2001). Pain signals reach the amygdala through the novel spino-ponto-amygdaloid pain-pathway (Bernard, Bester, & Besson, 1996; Gauriau & Bernard, 2002; Jasmin, Burkey, Card, & Basbaum, 1997) that connects pain centers in the spinal cord and brainstem to a particular part of the amygdala, the latero-capsular division of the central nucleus of the amygdala (CeA).

Importantly, this part of the amygdala (CeA) is critically involved in opioid and cannabinoid analgesia (Manning, 1998; Manning, Martin, & Meng, 2003) and is now designated as the "nociceptive amygdala" because of its high content of neurons that respond to painful events (Neugebauer & Li, 2002; Neugebauer & Li, 2003). These amygdala neurons serve other than classical sensory-discriminative functions: they are involved in the emotional responses to pain and exhibit a high degree of plasticity in a model of persistent pain (Neugebauer & Li, 2003;

Neugebauer, Li, Bird, Bhave, & Gereau, 2003). Inhibition of pain-related activity changes in the amygdala may be an important tool for the relief of pain and its emotional-affective component.

Management of Burn Pain

Despite pharmacological advances, successful management of both background and procedural pain associated with burn injuries remains a significant challenge. The perception of burn pain will vary according to the localization and degree of the injury, the stage of recovery in the healing process, and the child's previous experiences of pain and hospitalization. As discussed in the previous section, pain is complex with both cognitive and affective components heightening or lessening the perception of pain. In order to identify the most appropriate course of intervention, assessing pain must be the first step in understanding the child's pain response.

According to Martin-Herz, Thurber, and Patterson (2000), background pain and procedural pain vary according to intensity and duration with background pain generally lasting longer and procedural pain having greater intensity. Procedural burn pain (wound care, staple removal, debridement, and rehabilitation therapy) should be measured before, during and after the procedure. Background pain should be measured when the patient is at rest and no other procedure is occurring. Marvin (1995) provides a detailed description of pediatric pain measurement scales and recommends that the child's developmental level be considered. The music therapist's assessment of pain should include the following components: affective and cognitive responses, pain intensity and duration, previous coping strategies, developmental level, and observed parental interaction.

In their analysis of procedural pain, Martin-Herz et al. (2000) create an interesting continuum model ranging from avoidance to full participation in describing the coping preferences of children. It is important to determine if the child will be an active participant in the procedure or if the child wishes to completely focus attention away from the event. Sometimes, patients fall somewhere in-between the continuum and prefer to receive information during the procedure while simultaneously attending to a musical instrument.

Music therapy interventions can be applied systematically according to the child's coping style and tendency to avoid or approach the painful stimulus. Ideally, the music therapy process should begin at least 10 minutes prior to the procedure and continue after the procedure has finished. The contextual support model of music therapy (Robb, 2000) presents a versatile technique, active music engagement, which targets both the affective and cognitive components of pain. According to Thurber, Martin-Herz, and Patterson (2000), the child's perception of control over the event can be a significant factor in procedural coping. The music therapist can offer the patient choices of instruments to play and songs to sing while also facilitating communication between the patient and staff person performing the procedure. Turry (1997) describes an improvisational approach that integrates the process of what his happening during the procedure within the structure and lyrics of the music. Active music engagement, incorporating improvisation, can support the patient by offering control, validating feelings and processing of the experience:

L., an 8-year-old girl, needed several staples removed from her right hand. Music therapy was referred due to L.'s history of becoming increasingly fearful and combative during procedures. Prior to the procedure, L. chose to play the drum with her left hand while she practiced keeping her right hand still. The patient verbally initiated when she was ready to have her staples removed and pointed to the staple she wanted removed first. As the nurse removed each staple, L. played a steady rhythm on the drum and joined in the music therapist's rhythmic improvised singing, "goodbye staple, we don't need you." L. and the music therapist sang this phrase with each staple removed. L.'s affect remained positive. After all the staples were removed, L. ended the improvisation by singing about how she could now better use her right hand to do the things she enjoyed.

For patients who prefer an avoidance coping style, music has been used as a successful distraction technique (Fauerbach, Lawrence, Haythornthwaite, & Richter, 2002; Han, 1998; Herndon, 2002; Prensner, Yowler, Smith, Steele, & Fratianne, 2001). The following case illustrates how active music listening can be used to engage the child's attention away from a procedure:

K. was a 10-year-old girl receiving suture and staple removal from her right ear which necessitated her having to remain still throughout the procedure. K. was encouraged to focus her attention to an improvised melody played on the flute by the music therapy intern. The music therapist then verbally engaged the patient in a relaxation and imagery exercise. The flute music was improvised according to the thematic content of the story and provided a soothing and melodic accompaniment. The procedure was completed with minimal patient distress.

In providing procedural support to patients, clinicians must recognize the individuality of each patient. A strategy that is successful for one child may be inappropriate for another patient. As music therapists, it is important to know when not to use music, as in cases when the patient's distress has escalated and the music becomes an aversive stimulus. Also, in large burns where the debridement procedure can last 1 to 2 hours, it is important to recognize when coping skills become exhausted. In these circumstances, offering the patient a variety of coping techniques throughout the duration of the procedure may be a necessary tactic.

Background or ongoing burn pain may be related to inflammation of the tissue, post-operative pain, or pain associated with the skin's healing process (Herndon, 2002). Using music therapy techniques that address the affective and cognitive components of pain should be utilized. Barrera, Rykov, and Doyle (2002) found that pediatric cancer patients had improved mood after an interactive music therapy session. These children also showed an improvement in their play performance after the music therapy session was completed. Loss of interest in play may be a sign of depression in children, particularly when there exists physical restriction due to illness or injury (Mahaney, 1990). Active music engagement, developmental musical play, active music listening, and therapeutic songwriting are all effective techniques for coping with pain and anxiety issues.

On the burn ICU, the ability of patients to actively engage in music activities will vary according to developmental level, location of injury, degree of alertness, and physical endurance. For coping with background pain, music therapy goals may include increasing time duration the patient attends to music activities, increasing independent participation, increasing opportunity for choice and control, improving positive affect, and decreasing negative self-statements and perceptions. The following case example demonstrates how music therapy can facilitate coping with ongoing pain issues:

J. was a 10-year-old boy from Mexico who was recovering from a 45% total-body-surface-area burn to his lower extremities. During music therapy sessions, J. often chose various instruments to play as he and the music therapist improvised various songs about his hospitalization experience. During one particular session, J. played the keyboard as the music therapist accompanied him on the guitar. A call-response style song improvisation began to unfold with J. singing about his pain. The music therapist supported J. by singing about how far along he had come in his recovery. He then continued to sing and create lyrics about his skin healing and his upcoming discharge home.

In working with children in pain, it is important to validate the patient's response to pain while also reappraising the experience. For example, during debridement it is important for the patient to understand that cleaning the wounds helps heal the skin and minimizes the risk for infection. If the patient has a negative perception and views the pain as punishment, it can lead to feelings of guilt and helplessness, which can then exacerbate the pain response (Martin-Herz et al., 2000).

Pain is a part of the burn healing process. However, experiencing pain on a long-term basis can have adverse effects such as development of anxiety, depression and stress-related disorders (Huyser & Parker, 1999; Stoddard et al., 2002). Applying our knowledge of pain mechanisms and the components involved, music therapists can have an important role in helping patients through the recovery process.

TRAUMA

Traumatology is a developing field that can provide clinicians with valuable insight into the potential harmful effects of trauma on the neurological development of children. Neuroimaging studies on childhood trauma and posttraumatic stress disorder (PTSD) have shown frontal lobe abnormalities, decreased intracranial and cerebral volumes, and attenuated development in the hippocampus and amygdala compared with control groups (Carrion et al., 2001; De Bellis et al., 1999; Teicher et al., 2003). According to Perry, Pollard, Blakley, Baker, and Vigilante (1995), early childhood experiences directly influence how information is organized and synthesized into the developing brain. When the body enters a prolonged state of stress and hyperarousal, adverse neurological effects may occur. The likelihood of detrimental effects on the child's neurological functioning is positively correlated with the duration of the traumatic experience (Perry et al., 1995). Teicher, Anderson, Polcari, Anderson, and Navalta (2002) further add that these changes in brain structure increase the risk of psychiatric disorders such as depression, borderline personality, attention-deficit disorder, substance abuse, and posttraumatic stress disorder.

In addition to the actual event of the injury, recovering from a severe burn can be an ongoing traumatic experience in itself. Prolonged hospitalization, separation from family and home, recurrent and continued painful medical procedures, physical helplessness, and multiple losses often lead to symptoms of acute stress disorder (Daviss, Racusin, et al., 2000; Wintgens, Boileau, & Robaey, 1997). Herndon (2002) also states that both acute stress disorder and PTSD are considerable consequences in survivors of severe burn injury. Symptoms include nightmares, intrusive thoughts, flashbacks of the event, altered sleep patterns, flat affect, memory problems, social withdrawal, poor concentration, and exaggerated startle response (Daviss, Racusin, et al.,

2000; Herndon, 2002; Robert, Blakeney, Villareal, Rosenberg, & Meyer, 1999). However, the brain processes and integrates both the traumatic incident and the therapeutic intervention, thus having the potential to positively enhance emotional and cognitive development (Perry et al., 1995).

The clinical implications of traumatology are also important for music therapists. As delineated by Sears (1968), music as a therapeutic modality offers an experience within structure, self-organization, and relating to others. Each of these constructs in music therapy can directly impact those areas adversely affected by trauma. The music therapy experience can offer traumatized children an opportunity to have structure, control, and organization in the hospital environment, can offer a safe outlet for self-expression, and provide a means of positive interpersonal interaction. As previously mentioned in this chapter, the contextual support model of music therapy (Robb, 2000) can also be applicable in helping the burned child cope with the trauma experience. This model has the necessary components (structure, autonomy, and involvement) to counter the potential developmental problems that put the burn-injured child at risk.

Addressing concerns related to coping with trauma should begin on the intensive care unit. The assessment process should include observing the child's ability to make decisions, ability to interpersonally engage, affective response, developmental level of functioning, and possible trauma reactions such as increased startle response and hypervigilance. Singing songs familiar to the patient and providing musical play at the child's bedside can provide safety and comfort in an environment surrounded by aversive stimulation. Active music engagement is a technique most often used at this stage of recovery. However, physical limitations caused by severe burns can hinder functioning and present a challenge in identifying ways for patients to be independent and have control in their environment. Creativity in engaging the patient is a necessary skill for the music therapist. The following case example illustrates the application of active music engagement when physical limitations are a significant obstacle:

> *M. was a 12-year-old girl who was initially treated for four months at a hospital in South America prior to her transfer to this facility. Her 19-year-old brother accompanied the patient as her legal guardian and caretaker. Due to the localization of her injuries and recent surgical procedures, M., initially, had complete restriction of movement in all extremities. Upon assessment, M. was verbally withdrawn, made minimal eye contact, had flat affect, and was grieving the loss of her fingers as well as the death of her father from the accident. Music therapy goals included increasing verbal interaction and positive affect. During the session, the music therapist brought and demonstrated various melodic and percussive instruments at M.'s bedside. With encouragement, M. began to choose instruments for the music therapist and her brother to play. M. then directed musical improvisations by verbally indicating tempo, dynamics and cueing when to start and stop playing. During the sessions, M.'s verbalizations increased and she began to smile spontaneously in response to hearing her musical creations. Later in her treatment, M. attended group music therapy where she was able to identify with other children her age that had similar physical limitations. Toward the end of her hospitalization, M. became a peer group leader, initiated volunteering for*

activities and demonstrated ways to be independent in playing instruments with her physical challenges.

Therapeutic songwriting is another technique that has been used to aid the emotional recovery process for burn and trauma patients. Robb (1996) described decreased feelings of helplessness and increased coping skills as added benefits of this intervention for traumatically injured adolescents. Therapeutic songwriting ranges from word substitutions to complete original compositions and can be easily adapted according to the child's developmental status. For burn patients, common issues expressed in the lyrics have included feelings of anger and helplessness, pain associated with debridement, rehabilitation procedures, desire for independence, and interactions with hospital staff (Tuden, Bishop, & Herndon, 1998). Edwards (1998) comments that the song structure can provide a context for understanding the patients' daily treatments and offer a sense of control in their recovery process. With permission from the patients/songwriters, completed songs can be made available to other patients as a means to share experiences and decrease feelings of isolation. Using songwriting in this way can be a powerful therapeutic tool in helping patients identify and express thoughts and feelings articulated through the song's lyrics.

The burn-injured child may not be the only one affected by trauma. Perry et al. (1995) state that the child's hyperarousal response can be exacerbated or lessened by the level of the caregiver's alarm state. Therefore, the music therapist should maintain a calm presence when working on the intensive care unit and provide emotional support to the child's caregiver when necessary. Music therapy can strengthen the connection among family members by enhancing non-stressful and emotionally supportive interactions during sessions (McDonnell, 1984). A more detailed discussion about parental involvement in the music therapy process occurs later in this chapter.

REHABILITATION

A rigorous physical and occupational therapy program is an essential part of the child's treatment in order to attain better functional outcomes. Rehabilitation protocols begin immediately upon hospital admission and are implemented according to the severity and location of the burns. Part of the rehabilitation process consists of positioning and splinting the patient as a method to prevent contractures, and limb deformities and facilitate improved function (Herndon, 2002). The other major aspect of burn rehabilitation is the aggressive exercise component, which includes passive and active range of motion exercises, ambulation, stretching, strengthening, endurance training, and purposeful activities (Herndon, 2002). It is in this realm where the music therapist can provide complementary treatment to enhance the overall physical rehabilitation process for pediatric burn patients.

Information on the application of music therapy in pediatric burn rehabilitation is sparse. Rudenberg and Royka (1989) provide some explanation about the role music can have in reinforcing rehabilitative goals and encouraging active range of motion through motivating music activities. The authors emphasize that music therapists must have awareness in choosing and positioning instruments for patients in order to provide the most successful experience.

In choosing protocols for music therapy in rehabilitation, the Neurologic Music Therapy (NMT) model (Thaut, 1999) provides the most evidence-based approach. Although its clinical applications have primarily addressed neurological injuries and disorders, the basic principles of the NMT model can be applied to pediatric burn rehabilitation. The auditory and motor systems are interconnected (Thaut, Kenyon, Schauer, & McIntosh, 1999) such that rhythmic cues can facilitate motor planning and coordination. In burn rehabilitation, motor coordination is a significant element in active and functional exercise (Herndon, 2002). Thus, the standardized techniques of "Patterned Sensory Enhancement" and "Therapeutic Instrumental Music Playing" (Thaut, 1999) can be applied clinically with pediatric burn patients as part of their rehabilitation program.

The technique, Patterned Sensory Enhancement (PSE), uses the elements of music such as tempo, dynamic, and pitch to provide the spatial, temporal and force cues to direct functional movements (Thaut, 1999). These cues are specific to the movement patterns necessary for the patient to rehabilitate. In burn rehabilitation PSE can be applied during active exercise to facilitate the sequence and time duration for the movement tasks. For example, flexion and extension of fingers is a common exercise for patients with hand burns. Using a keyboard, the music therapist can play note clusters to cue the flexion phase, hold that note cluster to cue intensity and time duration, and then play an open chord to cue extension phase of the exercise. The following case example illustrates how PSE can be adapted using a child-oriented approach:

> *E., a 5-year-old boy from Mexico with an 86% total-body-surface-area burn, was reluctant to participate in physical therapy when it was time to work on standing and balancing. Using a traditional children's song from Mexico about elephants balancing on a spider web called "Los Elefantes," E. wore an elephant mask and pretended he was an elephant. As the physical therapist held and supported the patient to move and balance his body side to side, the music therapist played the guitar in 6/8 meter and sang with the patient. The meter and tempo cued the specific movements while the choice of song made the exercise motivating and enjoyable.*

Therapeutic Instrumental Music Playing (TIMP) is a technique that can be nicely tailored for pediatric burn patients engaging in functional exercises and purposeful activities. For burn patients, increasing endurance, strength and coordination via purposeful movement enhances independent participation in activities of daily living (Herndon, 2002). Thaut (1999) describes TIMP as the therapeutic application of instruments to stimulate functional movement patterns and "enhance range of motion, endurance, functional hand movements, finger dexterity, and limb coordination." Instruments are selected for the patient to play based upon the movements specified by the physical or occupational therapist. For example, to isolate the movement of elbow extension and flexion, a patient could strum an autoharp while the music therapist presses the chord buttons. It is important that the music therapist collaborate with the rehabilitation therapist to know the exact movement pattern to isolate.

For patients who have been on bed rest for an extended period of time, muscle weakness and atrophy can result (Herndon, 2002). TIMP can be used to improve endurance as patients work to regain their strength. This technique can be especially beneficial for patients positioned on a tilt table who require increased toleration of the upright position. While the patient is in the upright position, the music therapist can engage the child in TIMP activities to increase endurance of the upper extremities while simultaneously helping the patient cope with weight bearing on the lower extremities.

At times, the music therapist will have the dual purpose of providing coping skills for pain and anxiety as well as providing functional activities for enhancing fine and gross motor skills. For burn patients, pain is experienced with movement due to skin tightness and edema. However, Herndon (2002) states that the pain will decrease significantly with increased active movement since it stretches the skin and reduces swelling. Also, Melchert-McKearnan, Deitz, Engel, and White (2000) found better results for decreasing pain associated with movement when children engaged in purposeful activities versus routine exercises. The music therapist can integrate the coping techniques, mentioned previously in this chapter, into the child's rehabilitation sessions. For example, active music engagement can be combined simultaneously with TIMP as in the following case example:

> *Five-year-old D. had sustained a 94% total-body-surface-area burn with severe burns to both hands resulting in extensive rehabilitative needs. The music therapist was referred by the occupational therapist due to D.'s pain experienced while she received passive stretching exercises to her hands. During the session as the OT stretched her right hand, D. grasped a mallet with her left hand to play the drum and sing her favorite children's songs. As her pain increased, the music therapist began an improvised song using the words, "no more pain," while encouraging the child to strongly beat in rhythm on the drum. D.'s affect became more positive as she engaged in this improvisation while also maintaining a strong palmer grasp with her left hand for several minutes as she continued to play the drum.*

OTHER CLINICAL ISSUES

Respiratory Concerns

In the case of inhalation injury or other respiratory complications, a child treated for burns may require mechanical ventilation. Patients' levels of consciousness and alertness while on mechanical support will vary according to individual circumstances. Several studies have investigated music listening as a non-pharmacological treatment for anxiety for patients requiring ventilated assistance (Almerud & Petersson, 2003; Chlan, 1998; Wong, Lopez-Nahas, & Molassiotis, 2001). Each of these studies found music listening to be a cost-effective and beneficial intervention to facilitate relaxation for this population. Besides ventilation, Christenberry (1979) and Rudenberg and Royka (1989) recommend therapeutic singing, deep breathing, and playing wind instruments as methods to use with patients requiring improvement of lung capacity.

Music therapy research has not explored the influence music and rhythm may have on maintaining respiratory rate as patients are weaned or extubated from mechanical ventilation. In order for patients to be taken off mechanical ventilation, they need to be stable enough to support their own ventilatory needs such as maintaining respiration rate (Herndon, 2002). Haas, Distenfeld, and Axen (1986) revealed that musical rhythm could serve as a pacemaker to entrain respiration rate. Since respiration is primarily an involuntary function, using rhythmic respiratory entrainment should be used only as a supportive measure in helping patients to sustain breathing rate upon weaning or extubation. Rhythmic respiratory entrainment, using rhythm to support and facilitate the breathing patterns of patients being weaned from mechanical ventilation, involves the music therapist playing a rhythm matched to the patient's breathing rate before, during, and after the weaning procedure. This technique, observed clinically promising at this facility on a case-by-case basis, needs to be investigated to determine clinical effectiveness prior to becoming a standardized protocol. Furthermore, before addressing any respiratory issues, it is critical for the music therapist to consult with the respiratory therapist to determine the most appropriate application of music.

Developmental Considerations

The longer a child is hospitalized the more at risk he or she becomes for experiencing developmental delays. The length of stay for a severe burn injury can range from a few weeks to several months depending upon each unique case. Unfortunately, the effects of hospitalization and severe injury can be long-term. Gorga et al. (1999) found developmental problems more prevalent in pediatric burn survivors than physical or functional problems. They recommend that appropriate developmental activities be integrated into the child's recovery process as an integral component of treatment.

Music therapy has been used successfully in the pediatric medical setting to address developmental concerns in the areas of fine and gross motor skills, speech and language development, and socialization (Barrickman, 1989; Kennelly, 2000). On the burn unit, both individual and group music therapy sessions should be implemented to target developmental skills (Bishop et al., 1996). The music therapy assessment should include the child's developmental history and current level of functioning. On the intensive care unit, developmental goals can be simultaneously integrated into the treatment plan.

Group music therapy can also be an effective intervention for addressing social, motor, and cognitive skills within a normalized and nonthreatening environment (Tuden et al., 2000). Bishop et al. (1996) further adds that children may "be motivated to use extremities that they have avoided using due to pain and limitations" (p. 90). Encouraging patients to problem-solve physical challenges encountered during group music therapy can facilitate the adjustment process as they return to school, home, and the community.

Parental and Caregiver Involvement

A burn injury does not only affect the child but the entire family. In the intensive care unit environment, it is common for parents to feel overwhelmed, uncomfortable, out of control, or uncertain about how to speak or interact with their child. Research has shown a strong correlation between intensity of parental distress and the child's psychological adjustment (Daviss, Mooney, et al., 2000; LeDoux, Meyer, Blakeney, & Herndon 1998). Landolt, Grubenmann, and Meuli, (2002) found that healthy family relationships, versus burn size, scarring, or socioeconomic status, most predicted improved quality of life outcomes for pediatric burn survivors. The response of the parent can positively or negatively influence the child's coping behavior (Kirby & Whelan, 1996). Parental involvement, when combined with staff guidance and support, has even been shown to reduce pain perception in children undergoing invasive medical procedures on the burn unit (George & Hancock 1993). Including parents in their child's healing process can provide them with a sense of control and enhance their own coping strategies.

The music therapist should carefully observe parent–child interaction and keep parents informed about their child's music therapy treatment plan. In every session, the music therapist can model appropriate ways to interact and engage with the child and involve the parents according to their individual comfort levels. For example, the therapist can encourage the patient to select instruments for the parent to play or choose songs for the family to sing together at the child's bedside. Some parents choose to use the music therapy session for their own respite time while others prefer to participate. Because parents typically are the primary people in the child's life, it is vital that they are actively involved in the recovery process. However, as clinicians, we need to adjust our therapeutic interventions according to the different coping styles and family dynamics observed during treatment.

FUTURE IMPLICATIONS

In an effort to develop systematic protocols and improve outcomes for pediatric burn patients, it is critical that music therapists collaborate with research scientists from other disciplines. Increased understanding of the influence of music on the brain and limbic system in particular, on the emotional–affective and cognitive processing, and other physiological functions, will provide music therapists an evidence-based approach to validate clinical effectiveness. In support of an integrative "holistic" health care approach, music therapy can claim an ever increasing appreciation of its crucial role in pediatric burn care.

REFERENCES

Aggleton, J. P. (2000). *The amygdala: A functional analysis* (2nd ed.) Oxford: University Press.

Almerud, S., & Petersson, K. (2003). Music therapy—A complimentary treatment for mechanically ventilated intensive care patients. *Intensive & Critical Care Nursing, 19*(1), 21–30.

Barrera, M. E., Rykov, M. H., & Doyle, S. L. (2002). The effects of interactive music therapy on hospitalized children with cancer: A pilot study. *Psycho-Oncology, 11*(5), 379–388.

Barrickman, J. (1989). A developmental music therapy approach for preschool hospitalized children. *Music Therapy Perspectives, 7*, 10–16.

Basbaum, A. I. (1999). Distinct neurochemical features of acute and persistent pain. *Proceedings of the National Academy of Sciences of the United States of America, 96*, 7739–7743.

Becerra, L. R., Breiter, H. C., Stojanovic, M., Fishman, S., Edwards, A., Comite, A. R., & Gonzalez, R. G. (1999). Human brain activation under controlled thermal stimulation and habituation of noxious heat: An fMRI study. *Magnetic Resonance in Medicine, 41*, 1044–1057.

Bernard, J.-F., Bester, H., & Besson, J. M. (1996). Involvement of the spino-parabrachio-amygdaloid and -hypothalamic pathways in the autonomic and affective emotional aspects of pain. *Progress in Brain Research, 107*, 243–255.

Bingel, U., Quante, M., Knab, R., Bromm, B., Weiller, C., & Buchel, C. (2002). Subcortical structures involved in pain processing: Evidence from single-trial fMRI. *Pain, 99*, 313–321.

Bishop, B., Christenberry, A., Robb, S., & Rudenberg, M. T. (1996). Music therapy and child life interventions with pediatric burn patients. In M. A. Froehlich (Ed.), *Music therapy with hospitalized children: A creative arts child life approach* (pp. 87–108). Cherry Hill, NJ: Jeffrey Books.

Blood, A. J., & Zatorre, R. J. (2001). Intensely pleasurable responses to music correlate with activity in brain regions implicated in reward and emotion. *Proceedings of the National Academy of Sciences of the United States of America, 98*, 11818–11823.

Bonaz, B., Baciu, M., Papillon, E., Bost, R., Gueddah, N., Le Bas, J. F., Fournet, J., & Segebarth, C. (2002). Central processing of rectal pain in patients with irritable bowel syndrome: An fMRI study. *American Journal of Gastroenterology, 97*, 654–661.

Bornhovd, K., Quante, M., Glauche, V., Bromm, B., Weiller, C., & Buchel, C. (2002). Painful stimuli evoke different stimulus-response functions in the amygdala, prefrontal, insula and somatosensory cortex: a single-trial fMRI study. *Brain, 125*, 1326–1336.

Carrion, V. G., Weems, C. F., Eliez, S., Patwardhan, A., Brown, W., Ray, R. D., Reiss, A. L. (2001). Attenuation of frontal asymmetry in pediatric posttraumatic stress disorder. *Biological Psychiatry, 50*(12), 943–951.

Chlan, L. (1998). Effectiveness of a music therapy intervention on relaxation and anxiety for patients receiving ventilatory assistance. *Heart & Lung, 27*(3), 169–176.

Christenberry, E. B. (1979). The use of music therapy with burn patients. *Journal of Music Therapy, 16*(3), 138–148.

Daveson, B. (1999). A model of response: Coping mechanisms and music therapy techniques during debridement. *Music Therapy Perspectives. 17*(2), 92–98.

Daviss, W. B., Mooney, D., Racusin, R., Ford, J. D., Fleischer, A., McHugo, G. J. (2000). Predicting posttraumatic stress after hospitalization for pediatric injury. *Journal of the Academy of Child and Adolescent Psychiatry, 39*(5), 576–583.

Daviss, W. B., Racusin, R., Fleischer, A., Mooney, D., Ford, J. D., & McHugo, G. J. (2000). Acute stress disorder symptatology during hospitalization for pediatric injury. *Journal of the Academy of Child and Adolescent Psychiatry, 39*(5), 569–575.

De Bellis, M. D., Keshavan, M. S., Clark, D. B., Casey, B. J., Giedd, J. N., Boring, A. M., Frustaci, K., & Ryan, N. D. (1999). Developmental traumatology. Part II: Brain development. *Biological Psychiatry, 45*(10), 1271–1284.

Derbyshire, S. W. G., Jones, A. K. P., Gyulai, F., Clark, S., Townsend, D., & Firestone, L. L. (1997). Pain processing during three levels of noxious stimulation produces differential patterns of central activity. *Pain, 73*, 431–445.

Dubner, R., & Gold, M. (1999). The neurobiology of pain. *Proceedings of the National Academy of Sciences of the United States of America, 96*, 7627–7630.

Edwards, J. (1994). The use of music therapy to assist children who have severe burns. *The Australian Journal of Music Therapy, 5*, 3–6.

Edwards, J. (1995). "You are singing beautifully": Music therapy and the debridement bath. *The Arts in Psychotherapy, 22*(1), 53–55.

Edwards, J. (1998). Music therapy for children with severe burn injury. *Music Therapy Perspectives, 16*(2), 20–25.

Fauerbach, J. A., Lawrence, J. W., Haythornthwaite, J. A., & Richter, L. (2002). Coping with the stress of a painful medical procedure. *Behaviour Research and Therapy, 40*, 1003–1015.

Fields, H. L., & Basbaum, A. I. (1999). Central nervous system mechanisms of pain modulation. In P.D.Wall & R. Melzack (Eds.), *Textbook of pain* (pp. 309–329). London, UK: Churchill Livingstone.

Fratianne, R. B., Prensner, J. D., Huston, M. J., Super, D. M., Yowler, C. J., & Standley, J. M. (2001). The effect of music-based imagery and musical alternate engagement on the burn debridement process. *Journal of Burn Care & Rehabilitation, 22*(1), 47–53.

Gauriau, C., & Bernard, J.-F. (2002). Pain pathways and parabrachial circuits in the rat. *Experimental Physiology 87*, 251–258.

George, A., & Hancock, J. (1993). Reducing pediatric burn pain with parent participation. *Journal of Burn Care & Rehabilitation, 14*(1), 104–107.

Gorga, D., Johnson, J., Bentley, A., Silverberg, R., Glassman, M., Madden, M., Yurt, R., & Nagler, W. (1999). The physical, functional, and developmental outcome of pediatric burn survivors from 1 to 12 months postinjury. *Journal of Burn Care & Rehabilitation, 20*(2), 171–178.

Haas, F., Distenfeld, S., & Axen, K. (1986). Effects of perceived music rhythm on respiratory patterns. *Journal of Applied Physiology, 61*(3), 1185–1191.

Han, P. (1998). The use of music in managing pain for hospitalised children. *The Australian Journal of Music Therapy, 9,* 44–56.

Haythornthwaite, J. A., Sieber, W. J., & Kerns, R. D. (1991). Depression and the chronic pain experience. *Pain, 46,* 177–184.

Heinricher, M. M., & McGaraughty, S. (1999). Pain-modulating neurons and behavioral state. In R. Lydic & H. A. Baghdoyan (Eds.), *Handbook of behavioral state control* (pp. 487–503). New York: CRC Press .

Herndon, D. H. (Ed.). (2002). *Total burn care* (2nd ed.). London: W. B. Saunders.

Huyser, B. A., & Parker, J. C. (1999). Negative affect and pain in arthritis. *Rheumatic Diseases Clinics of North America, 25,* 105–121.

Jasmin, L., Burkey, A. R., Card, J. P., & Basbaum, A. I. (1997). Transneuronal labeling of a nociceptive pathway, the spino-(trigemino-)parabrachio-amygdaloid, in the rat. *Journal of Neuroscience, 17,* 3751–3765.

Kennelly, J. (2000). The specialist role of the music therapist in developmental programs for hospitalised children. *Journal of Pediatric Health Care, 14*(2), 56–59.

Kirby, R. J., & Whelan, T. A. (1996). The effects of hospitalisation and medical procedures on children and their families. *Journal of Family Studies, 2*(1), 65–77.

Landolt, M., Grubenmann, S., & Meuli, M. (2002). Family impact greatest: Predictors of quality of life and psychological adjustment in pediatric burn survivors. *Journal of Trauma, 53*(6), 1146–1151.

LeDoux, J., Meyer, W. J., III, Blakeney, P. E., & Herndon, D. N. (1998). Relationship between parental emotional states, family environment and the behavioral adjustment of pediatric burn survivors. *Burns, 24,* 425–432.

Loveszy, R. (1991). The use of Latin music, puppetry, and visualization in reducing the physical and emotional pain of a child with severe burns. In K. E. Bruscia (Ed.), *Case studies in music therapy* (pp. 153–161). Phoenixville, PA: Barcelona Publishers.

Mahaney, N. B. (1990). Restoration of play in a severely burned three-year-old child. *Journal of*

Burn Care & Rehabilitation, 11(1), 57–63.

Manning, B. H. (1998). A lateralized deficit in morphine antinociception after unilateral inactivation of the central amygdala. *Journal of Neuroscience, 18,* 9453–9470.

Manning, B. H., Martin, W. J., & Meng, I. D. (2003). The rodent amygdala contributes to the production of cannabinoid-induced antinociception. *Neuroscience, 120,* 1157–1170.

Martin-Herz, S. P., Thurber, C. A., & Patterson, D. R. (2000). Psychological principles of burn wound pain in children. II: Treatment applications. *Journal of Burn Care & Rehabilitation, 21*(5), 458–472.

Marvin, J. A. (1995). Pain assessment versus management. *Journal of Burn Care & Rehabilitation, 16*(3), 348–357.

McDonnell, L. (1984). Music therapy with trauma patients and their families on a pediatric service. *Music Therapy, 4*(1), 55–63.

McGaraughty, S., & Heinricher, M. M. (2002). Microinjection of morphine into various amygdaloid nuclei differentially affects nociceptive responsiveness and RVM neuronal activity. *Pain, 96,* 153–162.

Meagher, M. W., Arnau, R. C., & Rhudy, J. L. (2001). Pain and emotion: Effects of affective picture modulation. *Psychosomatic Medicine, 63,* 79–90.

Melchert-McKearnan, K., Deitz, J., Engel, J. M., & White, O. (2000). Children with burn injuries: Purposeful activity versus rote exercise. *The American Journal of Occupational Therapy, 54*(4), 381–390.

Neugebauer, V. (2002). Metabotropic glutamate receptors—Important modulators of nociception and pain behavior. *Pain, 98,* 1–8.

Neugebauer, V., & Li, W. (2002). Processing of nociceptive mechanical and thermal information in central amygdala neurons with knee-joint input. *Journal of Neurophysiology, 87,* 103–112.

Neugebauer, V., & Li, W. (2003). Differential sensitization of amygdala neurons to afferent inputs in a model of arthritic pain. *Journal of Neurophysiology, 89,* 716–727.

Neugebauer, V., Li, W., Bird, G. C., Bhave, G., & Gereau, R. W. (2003). Synaptic plasticity in the amygdala in a model of arthritic pain: Differential roles of metabotropic glutamate receptors 1 and 5. *Journal of Neuroscience, 23,* 52–63.

Ohayon, M. M., & Schatzberg, A. F. (2003). Using chronic pain to predict depressive morbidity in the general population. *Archives of General Psychiatry, 60,* 39–47.

Paulson, P. E., Casey, K. L., & Morrow, T. J. (2002). Long-term changes in behavior and regional cerebral blood flow associated with painful peripheral mononeuropathy in the rat. *Pain, 95,* 31–40.

Perry, B. D., Pollard, R. A., Blakley, T. L., Baker, W. L., & Vigilante, D. (1995). Childhood trauma, the neurobiology of adaptation, and "use-dependent" development of the brain: How "states" become "traits." *Infant Mental Health Journal, 16*(4), 271–291.

Prensner, J. D., Yowler, C. J., Smith, L. F., Steele, A. L., & Fratianne, R. B. (2001). Music therapy for assistance with pain and anxiety management in burn treatment. *Journal of Burn Care & Rehabilitation, 22*(1), 83–88.

Rhudy, J. L., & Meagher, M. W. (2000). Fear and anxiety: Divergent effects on human pain thresholds. *Pain, 84,* 65–75.

Robb, S. L. (1996). Techniques in song writing: Restoring emotional and physical well being in adolescents who have been traumatically injured. *Music Therapy Perspectives, 14*(1), 30–37.

Robb, S. L. (2000). The effect of therapeutic music interventions on the behavior of hospitalized children in isolation: Developing a contextual support model of music therapy. *Journal of Music Therapy, 37*(2), 118–146.

Robb, S. L., Nichols, R. J., Rutan, R. L., Bishop, B. L., & Parker, J. C. (1995). The effects of music-assisted relaxation on preoperative anxiety. *Journal of Music Therapy, 32,* 2–21.

Robert, R., Blakeney, P. E., Villarreal, C., Rosenberg, L., & Meyer, W. J. (1999). Imipramine treatment in pediatric burn patients with symptoms of acute stress disorder: A pilot study. *Journal of the American Academy of Child & Adolescent Psychiatry, 38*(7), 873–882.

Rudenberg, M. T., & Royka, A. M. (1989). Promoting psychosocial adjustment in pediatric burn patients through music therapy and child life therapy. *Music Therapy Perspectives, 7,* 40–43.

Schneider, F., Habel, U., Holthusen, H., Kessler, C., Posse, S., Muller-Gartner, H. W., & Arndt, J. O. (2001). Subjective ratings of pain correlate with subcortical-limbic blood flow: An fMRI study. *Neuropsychobiology, 43,* 175–185.

Sears, W. W. (1968). Processes in music therapy. In E. T. Gaston (Ed.), *Music in therapy* (pp. 30–44). New York: Macmillan.

Stoddard, F. J., Sheridan, R. L., Saxe, G. N., King, B. S., King, B. H., Chedekel, D. S., Schnitzer, J. J., & Martyn, A. J. (2002). Treatment of pain in acutely burned children. *Journal of Burn Care & Rehabilitation, 23*(2), 135–156.

Stucky, C. L., Gold, M. S., & Zhang, X. (2001). Mechanisms of pain. *Proceedings of the National Academy of Sciences of the United States of America, 98,* 11845–11846.

Tarnowski, K. J. (Ed.). (1994). *Behavioral aspects of pediatric burns.* New York: Plenum Press.

Teicher, M. H., Anderson, S. L., Polcari, A., Anderson, C. M., & Navalta, C. P. (2002). Developmental neurobiology of childhood stress and trauma. *Psychiatric Clinics of North America, 25*(2), 397–426.

Teicher, M. H., Anderson, S. L., Polcari, A., Anderson, C. M., Navalta, C. P., & Kim, D. M. (2003). The neurobiological consequences of early stress and childhood maltreatment. *Neuroscience & Biobehavioral Reviews, 27*(1-2), 33–44.

Thaut, M. H. (1999). *Training manual for neurologic music therapy.* Fort Collins, CO: Center for Biomedical Research, Colorado State University.

Thaut, M. H., Kenyon, G. P., Schauer, M. L., & McIntosh, G. C. (1999). The connection between rhythmicity and brain function: Implications for movement disorders. *IEEE Engineering in Medicine and Biology, 18,* 101–108.

Thurber, C. A., Martin-Herz, S. P., & Patterson, D. R. (2000). Psychological principles of burn wound pain in children. I: Theoretical framework. *Journal of Burn Care & Rehabilitation, 21*(4), 376–387.

Tuden, C., Amrhein, C., Rosenberg, L., Sanford, A., Cucuzzo, N., & Herndon, D. N. (2000, March). *"Thank you for the music": Group music therapy for pediatric burn patients and their families.* Poster session presented at the annual meeting of the American Burn Association, Las Vegas, NV.

Tuden, C., Bishop, B., & Herndon, D. N. (1998, March). *Musical inspirations: Songwriting as a projective technique for pediatric burn survivors.* Poster session presented at the annual meeting of the American Burn Association, Chicago, IL.

Turry, A. (1997). The use of clinical improvisation to alleviate procedural distress in young children. In J. V. Loewy (Ed.), *Music therapy and pediatric pain* (pp. 89–96). Cherry Hill, NJ: Jeffrey Books.

Willis, W. D. (2002). Long-term potentiation in spinothalamic neurons. *Brain Research Reviews, 40,* 202–214.

Wintgens, A., Boileau, B., & Robaey, P. (1997). Posttraumatic stress symptoms and medical procedures in children. *Canadian Journal of Psychiatry, 42,* 611–616.

Wong, H. L., Lopez-Nahas, V., & Molassiotis, A. (2001). Effects of music therapy on anxiety in ventilator-dependent patients. *Heart & Lung, 30*(5), 376–387.

Wood, J. N., & Perl, E. R. (1999). Pain. *Current Opinion in Genetics and Development, 9,* 328–332.

Woolf, C. J., & Salter, M. W. (2000). Neuronal plasticity: increasing the gain in pain. *Science, 288,* 1765–1769.

Yaksh, T. L., Hua, X. Y., Kalcheva, I., Nozaki-Taguchi, N., & Marsala, M. (1999). The spinal biology in humans and animals of pain states generated by persistent small afferent input. *Proceedings of the National Academy of Sciences of the United States of America, 96,* 7680–7686.

ACKNOWLEDGMENTS

We would like to thank the Child Life Department at Shriners Burns Hospital-Galveston, Texas for integrating and promoting music therapy services into their dynamic program. We would also like to recognize the many young burn survivors who have so bravely endured the challenge of recovery and helped enlighten the process of music therapy in pediatric burn care.

V.N.'s work is supported by John Sealy Memorial Endowment Fund for Biomedical Research 2521-04 and NIH grant NS38261.

Four

∽

Critical Care: Clinical Applications of Music for Children on Mechanical Ventilation

Janice W. Stouffer, MT-BC
Beverly Shirk, RN, BSN, CCRN

INCREASINGLY, music is being applied to treatment of children in the critical care setting. Literature from the fields of both music therapy and healthcare support a wide range of therapeutic uses for music across all ages in the general medical setting. Studies conducted in the critical, or intensive, care setting have focused primarily on adults and neonates, and minimally on children. In particular, there is a lack of research aimed at addressing the needs of children who require mechanical ventilation in the critical care unit. Attempts on the part of healthcare professionals to incorporate music into treatment have raised a positive awareness of music therapy. However, with a few exceptions, methods and procedures have not always been the most therapeutic or guided by principles established in the music therapy literature. Similarly, a number of investigations conducted by music therapists alone have been limited in scientific rigor, and even in the provision of precise descriptions of methods and treatment protocols. Collaborative efforts between the two fields are beginning to emerge that will set the stage for significant advancement of knowledge regarding effective applications of music in the medical setting.

Of immediate concern to pediatric critical care providers is the impact of scientifically tested music protocols on physiological outcomes and requirements for sedation. Of no less importance is the role that music therapy plays in the psychological well being of the patients and their families. Children in the pediatric critical care unit (PCCU) often require assistive ventilation during the critical phase of illness or injury. Many require sedative medications to increase cooperation with procedures. Patients exhibit stress responses related to both physiologic disease processes and emotional reactions. Administration of sensory altering medications and intermittent sleep deprivation are contributing stressors as well. For those children who are alert and aware, the environment in the PCCU and the procedures experienced may cause increased fear, anxiety, and agitation. Ultimately, these physiological and emotional stressors produce deleterious changes in heart rate, respiratory rate and work of breathing, blood pressure, and oxygen saturation. Managing children requires careful attention not only to medical needs, but also to developmental stages and individual emotional responses. Research-based music treatment protocols have the ability to address this constellation of physiological and psychosocial needs by means that are both nonpharmacological and highly cost effective.

PEDIATRIC CRITICAL CARE

Diagnostic Conditions

Children admitted to the PCCU have sustained a life threatening injury or illness that may involve one or more of the major body systems. Patients often undergo invasive and technological procedures and are managed with carefully titrated medications. This means that the medications administered are increased or decreased according to the child's physical responses observed at any given moment. As a result, these patients require constant hemodynamic and respiratory monitoring, often with a 1:1 or 2:1 patient to staff ratio. Critically ill children typically have respiratory compromise as a primary or secondary process. A wide array of medical and surgical or traumatic etiologies may be involved (see Table 1).

Table 1
Pediatric Critical Injuries/Illnesses

Medical	**Surgical**	**Trauma**
Pneumonia	Neurosurgery	Near-drowning
Meningitis	Cardio thoracic surgery	Head injury (minor–severe)
Septic shock	Airway manipulations	Chest injury (blunt–penetrating)
Newborn apnea	Spinal surgery	Liver injury
Hematologic crisis	Lung surgery	Spleen injury
Multiple organ dysfunction	Extra corporeal membrane oxygenation (ECMO)	Orthopedic fracture and/or amputation
Severe asthma exacerbation	Renal transplantation	Spinal fracture
Diabetic keto acidosis	Cardiac transplantation	Spinal cord injury
Hepatic failure		Renal injury
Status epilepticus		Burns

Environmental Conditions

The CCU environment warrants special consideration. In general throughout many CCUs, levels of background sound are typically intensive. Movements around the unit are often urgent and fast-paced. Bedside equipment such as cardiac monitors, ventilators, and intravenous or enteral pumps are usually programmed to alarm loudly, alerting staff to potential problems. Measurements of background noise have been found to average 50–60 decibels (dB), with alarms increasing the levels up to 90 dB intermittently (Byers & Smyth, 1997). These measurements are comparable to those found in the environment for normal urban traffic and street activity. Figure 1 summarizes sounds typically found in this setting.

- Staff conversations (various intensity levels)
- Monitor alarms: ECG, IV, feeding pumps, ventilators
- Individual pager alarms
- Situational peaks around procedures and emergencies
- Medication cart and door alarms, sounds of opening/closing
- Supply doors and drawers opening/closing
- Patients and parents crying
- Telephones
- Overhead paging system alerts
- Charts, clipboards and binder notebooks opening/closing

Figure 1. *CCU Environmental Sounds* (Cabrera & Lee, 2000)

Space around the bed is limited due to the amount of equipment. Families have restricted access to their child as a result, and may also be confined to structured visitations around procedures or individual unit policies. Physical space limits must be anticipated as music therapists plan treatment interventions. Before approaching the patient in the PCCU, therapists must consult with bedside staff to determine an appropriate treatment plan. Level of desired sedation and the child's responses to stimulation or procedures should be considered. Particular attention should be directed to bedside equipment like monitor wires, intravenous lines, enteral feeding lines, drainage tubes, catheters, and ventilator tubing. Maintaining proper patient positioning may be critical in the individual child's care. Mobility limitations due to surgical or traumatic injuries may also impact the treatment plan.

Effects of Noise

Prior to addressing issues related to the application of music for desired outcomes, consideration must be given to the effects of background noise on stress responses. In a review of studies related to noise pollution in health care settings, Cabrera and Lee (2000) reported sound levels in various areas of hospitals to be 10 to 47dB higher than the recommendation of 45dB during the daytime made by both the Environmental Protection Agency and the International Noise Council. Areas tested included both operating rooms and intensive care units. These findings are significant in light of the elevating effect noise has been shown to have on blood pressure (McLean & Tarnopolsky, 1977), vasoconstrictor Angiotensin II (Dengerink, Wright, Thompson, & Dengerink, 1982), and serum cholesterol and triglyceride levels in Type A personality patients (Lovallo & Pishkin, 1980). A report involving normal school children documented lower problem solving scores, higher blood pressure, increased irritability and aggressiveness, and fatigue in response to continuous noise (Monroe, 1996). Negative, stressful effects of loud noises on the critically ill child, including talking, laughing, and music that is too loud or fast, are emphasized in nursing literature (Lewandowski 1992). Cabrera and Lee (2000) advocate not only for music therapy, but also a hospital Department of Sound to first control for and mask extraneous noise, then to develop treatment protocols applying appropriate music for specific patient populations.

Critical Needs of Children on Mechanical Ventilation

Mechanical ventilation is used to stabilize and treat respiratory failure, which is common in critically ill infants and children. Children are intubated through the mouth or nose into the trachea with an artificial airway connected to a mechanical ventilator. The machine is programmed to mimic normal respiratory patterns and oxygenation. With regard to medical treatment goals, patients may receive a high level of control of ventilation or may be able to participate with spontaneous breathing above the ventilator. Frequent analysis of the patient's respiratory effort and serum oxygenation is completed to determine respiratory effectiveness and guide further adjustments of machine settings. Children who require ventilation, as well as their families, are exposed to many unfamiliar sights, sounds and painful procedures while in the PCCU. Suctioning of mucous secretions, turning and changes of body position, and providing oral care or wound care may be necessary on a frequent basis around the clock. Staff utilize pharmacologic and nonpharmacologic measures to manage these experiences. Nursing treatment goals are centered around controlling deleterious behaviors such as attempting to sit up or pulling at life-sustaining tubes, maximizing comfort, and minimizing complications.

Traditional nonpharmacologic measures commonly used by nursing staff to promote comfort include environmental adaptations involving tactile, visual, and auditory experiences. Attention to avoiding extremes in temperature through radiant external warmers and blankets can minimize shivering or sweating, thereby increasing overall comfort. Patients are repositioned frequently to maintain skin integrity and maximize normal sensations. Infants, for example, may be comforted simply by swaddling in a blanket. An older child may find comfort in seeing or feeling familiar objects like a favorite toy or blanket. Whenever possible, staff should engage and empower parents to mimic normal patterns of comforting measures. During periods of family involvement, careful monitoring of environmental sounds must be included to avoid eliciting startle responses while assisting parents to talk or sing and touch their child as they would normally do at bedtime or naptime. Constant vigilance and reassessment of the child's clinical status is crucial to assure effective outcomes (Hazinski, 1992).

Sedation Side Effects

Sedative medications are generally used to maximize comfort for patients undergoing unpleasant procedures while maintaining adequate cardiorespiratory function. In children especially, the use of sedation increases compliance with care, in addition to decreasing pain and anxiety (Curley, Smith, and Moloney-Harmon, 1996; Hazinski, 1992). However, the use of sedative and analgesic medications has inherent risks which are summarized in Table 2.

Table 2
Effects of Sedation and Analgesic Medication

Category	**Effects and Considerations**
Over sedation	• Patient unable to participate in ventilator weaning, may lead to prolonged duration of mechanical ventilation and subsequently higher risk of infections, barotraumas. • More likely in a patient with liver/renal dysfunction.
Under sedation	• Child may feel scared or in pain • Can lead to premature self-extubation (with associated hypoxia or airway structural damage), agitation, respiratory variances, stimulation of stress response (immunosuppression, hypercoagulapathy, tachycardia)
Hemodynamic variances	• Tachycardia, hypotension, peripheral vasodilation • More prevalent in hypovolemic patients
Respiratory variances	• Increased work of breathing and metabolic/oxygenation demands, hypoxia, respiratory depression
Gastrointestinal variances	• Nausea, vomiting, constipation, and ileus • More prevalent with narcotic usage
Tolerance	• Occurs with prolonged usage • Withdrawal may follow if discontinued rapidly

In adult populations, the daily interruption of sedation infusions is utilized to guide neurologic injury management and is theorized to decrease duration of mechanical ventilation and CCU length of stay. Children have been less responsive to this process largely related to developmental inabilities to understand treatment rationales (Curley et al., 1996; Hazinski, 1992). A child who is suddenly wakened may exhibit stress behaviors like increases in heart rate, respiratory rate, crying, pulling at wires or tubes, or attempting to sit up. Titration of sedation doses to the least amount with maximal effect has been more successful through the use of behavior measurement tools such as the Riker Sedation-Agitation tool (Riker, Fraser, & Cox, 1994) (see Appendix A). A recent study comparing 138 experimental subject patients to 147 control patients supports behavioral measurement of sedation levels. Brattebo et al. (2002) were able to demonstrate a decreased length of ventilated days and CCU length of stay in adult ventilated patients through the implementation of a sedation scoring system and sedation administration protocol. In this team approach, CCU physicians defined the desired level of sedation twice daily with subsequent nursing titration of sedation dosing according to established guidelines. Understanding the use of sedation tools and working collaboratively with the CCU team, music therapists have the ability to impact the management of patient sedation needs.

INDICATIONS FOR MUSIC THERAPY

Given the dynamic medical status of critically ill children, their unique and varied developmental needs, and the conditions of an intense, unfamiliar environment, treatment in the

PCCU can increase the stress response at a time when medical stability of vital signs is crucial (Lewandowski, 1992). Physicians use a variety of approaches to manage these variables, including protocols to determine sedation needs, as well as scales to document desired sedation level. As medical conditions improve, children are able to be weaned from pharmacological and technological interventions. Their ability to demonstrate positive coping behaviors and to remain calm during weaning becomes the focus of care. Music therapy, as a nonpharmacological intervention, is indicated to assist with the weaning process.

In terms of physiological processes, music therapy is generally indicated for those children who have required prolonged, high levels of sedative medications while on invasive machines, children with respiratory illness or injury requiring maintenance of a relaxed state, and children who must undergo frequent painful procedures. As dosages of sedation and analgesic are decreased, music can assist regulation through entrainment of heart rate and respiratory rate, relaxation of muscle tone, and decreased work of breathing which facilitates overall oxygenation.

Psychosocially, children emerging from a highly sedated or coma state and beginning to experience fear and anxiety will benefit from calming interaction with the music and therapist. Other children are consistently alert and aware but require prolonged admissions for medical treatment (i.e., resolution of infection issues or chest fluid drainage) or may be awaiting procedures such as heart transplants. Music therapy is indicated for self expression, emotional coping, and development of adapted meaningful leisure activity. Expanding the scope of care beyond the patients to their families, music therapy activities are indicated for parents and siblings as well. Many demonstrate limited coping abilities, high anxiety, or have limited experience with adapting interaction and communication styles to accommodate new, atypical needs of their children. Ultimately, the degree to which the family can adjust and cope with the critical care needs and surroundings of the patient effects the child's well-being and potential for healing. Methods for best practice in the PCCU involve music therapists being prepared to address both the biomedical and psychosocial needs of the pediatric patients.

One clinical review involving children in critical care focused on the physical and emotional needs of cardiac care patients (Dun, 1995). Music therapy sessions were reported to provide a normalizing effect on the environment, contact with a nonmedical experience, positive stimulation, and distraction. Emphasis was also placed on empowerment of families, and achievement of normal parent/child relations through interaction facilitated by the music.

The majority of investigations pertaining to music in pediatric critical care have addressed the needs of premature infants in neonatal intensive care units. A recent meta-analysis of these studies with neonates demonstrated a significant overall effect size of almost a standard deviation ($d = .83$) (Standley 2002). The report included a summary, according to number of weeks gestation, of age-specific clinical applications to guide music therapists and health care professionals. It is important to note, particularly in the care of critically ill children, that none of the research reviewed reported auditory-evoked seizures or any other negative side effects following exposure to controlled music interventions. Auditory-evoked seizures are rare and unrelated to the use of therapeutic music (Zifkin & Andermann 2001).

In the absence of PCCU studies, indications for the therapeutic use of music with the general pediatric population include reduction of preoperative anxiety (Chetta,1981), anxiety during cardiac catheterization (Caire & Erickson, 1986; Micci, 1984), and postsurgical pain (Steinke,

1991). Music has been used with children to alleviate apprehension and discomfort associated with bone marrow aspirations (Pfaff, Smith, & Gowan, 1989), and pain and anxiety associated with injections (Fowler-Kerry & Lander, 1987) and lumbar punctures (Rasco, 1992). Case studies of children with severe head injury point to the use of music as structured stimulation and orientation during the emergence from coma (Rosenfeld & Dun, 1999). The increased use of music with hospitalized children is reflected through the emergence of literature to direct the clinical use of music by various practitioners. For example, Klein and Winkelstein (1996) published a guide for pediatric nurse practitioners stressing the importance of considering developmental stages when selecting appropriate music interventions and outlining the indications for seeking consultation from professionals trained in music therapy.

PRIMARY TREATMENT GOALS

Primary treatment goals for children in critical care, particularly those on mechanical ventilation, are to increase calming and relaxation. The assessment and measurement of anxiety in mechanically ventilated patients can be particularly challenging. Given the current lack of studies with children, initial guidelines may be found in reports with adults and infants. Adult patients who required ventilatory assistance, but were not heavily sedated, reported significantly less anxiety and demonstrated decreased heart and respiratory rates over time with music intervention compared to those who had not listened to music (Chlan, 1998). In a case study analysis using music therapy for mechanically ventilated infants immediately following suctioning, music seemed to increase sleep time, and decreased overall level of arousal and stress-related behaviors of some infants (Burke, Walsh, Oehler, & Gingras, 1995).

In a discussion of the use of nonpharmacologic approaches for patients receiving mechanical ventilation, Fontaine (1994) reinforced the critical need for more research to evaluate the effectiveness of music therapy interventions on patient responses in critical care settings. Passive music listening (to selections prepared by a trained music therapist) is favored over other approaches such as biofeedback or imagery because it requires less concentration on the part of critically ill patients with low energy states (Chlan & Tracy, 1999). Furthermore, therapeutic music audiotape sessions were more effective than a rest period in a study of acutely ill, mechanically ventilated adults. The patients reported less anxiety and were observed to be more relaxed during the music therapy sessions (Wong, Lopez-Nahas, & Molassiotis, 2001).

MUSIC AND SEDATION

Though sedation is highly indicated for patients receiving mechanical ventilation, a wide array of undesirable side effects have been documented (Chlan, 1998). Additionally, the stress of acute disease pathology combined with anxiety and fear perceptions during mechanical ventilation can lead to increased sympathetic nervous system symptomotology. The therapeutic use of music with this population has shown decreases in anxiety and enhancement of relaxation (Chlan, 2000).

In general, the sedating effects of music have been associated with a variety of favorable outcomes. Music can enhance the effects of analgesia in adult populations and reduce dosages of sedating agents (Tang et al., 1993; Tryba, 1996). In a single case study, music-assisted sedation was shown to decrease the number of asthma attacks and promote relaxation for an asthmatic patient in the perioperative phase of surgery (Ochiai, Okutani, Yoshimura, & Fu, 1995). Heitz, Symreng, and Scamman (1992) used music as audio analgesia. This investigation documented adult postoperative patients awakening to music as requiring less pain-relieving medication and waiting longer before requesting analgesics. Spintge (1989) summarized the results of controlled clinical studies involving more than 8,000 patients which showed that emotional relaxation by anxiolytic music was more effective than sedative drugs in controlling perioperative and postoperative anxiety. Usual dosages of sedative and analgesic drugs were reduced as much as 50% with music. Of clinical significance, a large majority of patients readily accepted this music treatment condition. In a two-phase study of patients requiring regional anesthesia during surgery, Koch, Kain, Ayoub, and Rosenbaum (1998) demonstrated that patients who listened to music used significantly less propofol to reach the same level of sedation as patients in the control group. Music also reduced the average opioid requirements by 44%. Lepage, Drolet, Girard, Grenier, and DeGagne (2001) studied patient-controlled midazolam usage in adults undergoing nononcologic spinal anesthesia. Patients who listened to music selections intraoperatively used less midazolam to achieve the same reported level of sedation. Nilsson, Rawal, Unestahl, Zetterberg, and Unosson (2001) noted that women undergoing elective hysterectomy who listened to music therapy audiotapes during surgery reported less postoperative pain and fatigue, and resumed activities faster than those who were exposed to routine operating room noise.

While many studies elucidate the promising effects of music used therapeutically to reduce the need for sedating agents and analgesics, further scientific rigor is needed to document its impact on requirements for these medications on critically ill infants and children. Important questions as to selection and type of music, method of presentation, and duration and frequency of presentation have yet to be answered.

SELECTION OF MUSIC

Among the most important variables to be considered in the development of a treatment protocol for critically ill children are methods for the selection of music. The therapeutic effect of music on sedation is directly related to the patient's preference for the music selections presented. This important determinant for the success of therapy is emphasized throughout the music therapy literature. Davis and Thaut (1989) suggest that "each individual may have a unique biological system that reacts to a given stimulus with an idiosyncratic but consistent physiological response and perceived psychological experience" (p.170). Their findings emphasized the need to consider music preference, familiarity with music, cultural context of the music, and past experiences, as well as perception of structure, dynamics and tempo in the music as important factors to selecting music for anxiety reduction and relaxation. Interestingly, Bonny (1986) identified a strong tendency among adult patients in a coronary care unit to report that preselected classical music had more relaxing properties than patient-selected popular music. She suggested that patients in a weakened or low energy state respond better to the relaxing properties of certain music than to familiar music which was in their repertoire of preferred tunes. Concurrently, empirical and evidenced-based information points to the enhanced effectiveness of therapeutic music when the properties of the selections coincide with a person's interest or appreciation for music compared to predetermined music selections (Christenberry, 1979; Gaston, 1968; Keller, 1995; Rider, 1997; Scartelli, 1989; Spintge, 1989).

While literature on adults is divided as to the merits of familiar, preferred music versus preselected "sedative" music, developmental considerations for children clearly point to the use of familiar, patient preferred music as being soothing and calming in the midst of an unfamiliar environment. Familiar music and recognizable melodies incorporated into the hospital setting offer a measure of safety and comfort for children (Kallay, 1997; Loewy, MacGregor, Richards, & Rodriquez, 1997). Additionally, the use of preferred music can re-establish a sense of control over an environment that may be stressful to a child (Davis, Gfeller, & Thaut, 1992). Typically, within the critical care setting, children are functionally unable or too young to communicate preferences. In this case, interview of the parent or primary caregiver provides necessary information as to music that previously has been shown to exert a calming effect, previous music experiences, or the music to which the child has been most exposed. Subsequent adaptation of the familiar melodies may then be done to produce a music selection that complies with accepted qualities of music for relaxation. Being able to account for the properties of "sedative" music while recognizing the benefits of considering patient background and music preference supports the need for individualized preparation of music selections.

Findings from a study conducted by Humpal (1998) serve as a starting point for determining preferences for music selections if parents and caregivers are unable to do so. Humpal surveyed music educators, music therapists, and educators involved with early childhood, and subsequently compiled a list of songs thought to be familiar and favored by children ages 6 and under. A comparison of these findings with a list of 42 songs reported by the Music Educators National Conference as being favorites of the general population in the United States revealed that only 25% of songs matched. The results of this investigation support the need to determine specific music preferences of children in this age group.

The role of the trained music therapist is to assess patient developmental needs and preferences, then to adapt the preferred selections according to guidelines for "sedative" music. Following a survey of the literature, Robb, Nichols, Rutan, Bishop, and Parker (1995) made several recommendations to guide the application of therapeutic music to decrease preoperative anxiety in children. These recommendations, summarized in Figure 2, may serve as a starting point for generalization to the critical care setting. It should be noted that, to date, surveys and guidelines established in the literature reflect properties and selections from mostly Western music literature. Cultural consideration must be given to these guidelines, particularly in regard to tonalities, rhythm, and phrasing if working with a more diverse population or patients who are more familiar with music other than traditional Western styles.

PRESENTATION OF MUSIC

Equally important to selection of music is the means by which it will be presented. Effective methods for music interventions have been cited in the literature. Studies of hospitalized children with cancer support the use of live, interactive therapeutic music interventions to illicit increased coping behaviors, increased comfort, and reduction in anxiety (Barrera, Rykov, & Doyle, 2002; Robb, 2000). Live music sessions have also proven effective as distraction and noninvasive pain

- Tempo of 60-70 beats per minute (bpm)
- Gradual and predictable dynamic changes
- Soft to moderately loud volume
- Regular rhythm without sudden tempo changes
- Sustained melodies in lower pitch range
- Consonant harmonies
- Music with soft tone qualities on strings, voice and piano

Figure 2. *Properties of Sedative Music*

management for pediatrics receiving intravenous starts, venipunctures, injections, and heel sticks (Malone, 1996). Children receiving the live musical interaction exhibited significantly fewer signs of behavioral distress than did a nonmusic control group.

While live interaction with the music therapist is usually most desirable, critical care conditions often warrant the use of recorded music selections. Treatments are typically required on a variable schedule, or on a PRN basis 24 hours per day. Recording live versions of songs chosen by the family allows for application of music treatment as needed, and ensures that music readily available to the nurses and families is consistently within parameters of sedative music as previously described. For purposes of empirical study, recording the adapted music ensures smooth transitions from song to song, allows use of the same instrumentation within subjects and across subjects, and therefore provides consistency of music presentation.

Additionally, due to environmental conditions such as machine noise, close proximity of beds with other patients and families, and continuous staff noise, use of headphones may be preferable to freefield music playing. Positive effects associated with the use of headphones to present audiotaped music include increased control over decibel level, attenuation of ambient noise, binaural presentation of stimuli, and delivery of music without effecting other patients on the unit (Cassidy & Ditty, 1998; Chlan & Tracy, 1999). The role of the music therapist is to determine the most effective method of presentation given the individual treatment objectives and environmental conditions.

Considerations for the presentation of adapted preferred music that has been recorded include monitoring of the volume level. Based on a survey of music presentation protocols with newborns and premature infants conducted by Cassidy and Ditty (1998), cassette or CD players should be calibrated by the audiology department, with volume being set at 60–80 dB. Volume controls need to be secured at this setting and checked regularly to control for purposeful or accidental adjustment by staff or family. Small, portable players are recommended for ease of placement. If battery operation is chosen, frequent monitoring of charge and use of rechargeable batteries is recommended.

DURATION AND FREQUENCY OF MUSIC INTERVENTION

Prescriptions for medical treatment are typically written in terms of dosage and frequency of administration. Laypersons who have experienced a positive personal change in response to certain music, whether for relaxation or stimulation, will frequently "self medicate," or use their music as needed, to bring about the desired effect. Within the medical setting, few studies involving music have addressed the issues of "how much" or "how often" music should be applied to achieve optimum effects. In reports that did specify length of treatment, the duration of audiotaped music applied for purposes of relaxation across various patient populations ranged between 20 to 30 minutes per presentation (Bailey, 1983; Bonny, 1983; Caine, 1991; Cassidy & Standley, 1995; Chlan, 1998, 2000; Guzzetta, 1995). No information regarding frequency, optimum schedule of treatment, or length of time between presentations was found. Music listening on a PRN basis may be administered following procedures such as suctioning, dressing changes, and changes of position in order to bring physiological and emotional responses back to a resting rate.

The wide variation in length and number of exposures to music across studies indicates the need for additional research to determine therapeutic levels regarding frequency, duration, and scheduling of music interventions. Attention to the amount of simultaneous bedside music and aural stimulation between interventions is warranted as well. Healthcare staff often require education as to the need for definitive periods of listening followed by periods of no music in order to avoid habituation. Well-meaning family members will often activate a continuous musical toy while a television and possibly even a tape or CD player are in operation. Overstimulation or habituation and tuning out of music altogether may quickly occur.

MUSIC AND MOTHER'S VOICE

Increasingly, hospitals are taking a more family-centered approach to the care of patients. Through education, parents are being involved in treatment planning, assisting with routine acute care procedures, and are prepared for the responsibility of long-term home care. Grasso, Button, Allison, and Sawyer (2000) studied caregivers of children between 4½ and 24 months of age with cystic fibrosis who required daily chest physiotherapy. After use of specifically composed and recorded music as an adjunct to this time consuming therapy, results showed significantly increased enjoyment of both children and parents in comparison with the control group who experienced both their regular routine and a placebo control of taped familiar music. A study of children in an emergency department setting assigned parents the critical responsibility of selecting the music that was most familiar to the child if the child was unable to communicate this information (Berlin, 1998). The investigators reported success in using this music to reduce behaviors consistent with pain and anxiety. Research with infants in a Neonatal Intensive Care Unit involved parent training in music and multimodal stimulation. Compared with controls, infants in the experimental group evidenced decreased stress behaviors while their parents demonstrated more appropriate actions and responses to the infants (Whipple, 2000).

More specifically, the impact of music and of mother's voice on pediatric patients has been investigated. Infants and preschool-age children were noted to fall asleep significantly sooner when they listened to lullabies, metronomes and/or recorded heartbeats than when they did not receive any auditory stimulation (Brackbill, Adams, Crowell, & Gray, 1966; Kagan & Lewis, 1965). In a study comparing the effects of music alone with mother's voice alone, Standley and Madsen (1990) observed that infants (age 2 to 8 months) listened more intensely to the music, and displayed fewer gross motor movements when presented with music stimulation alone. However, the duration of infant listening was longest for mother's voice. Neonates displayed changes in physiological measures, such as an increase in oxygen saturation levels and a decrease in oximeter alarms with music (Standley & Moore, 1995). When music stimuli were discontinued, these babies experienced a short period of depression in oxygen saturation levels. This response was not evident after exposure to mother's voice alone.

Because music alone and mother's voice alone exert positive effects on the physiological status of infants, it may be possible that a combination of mother's voice (or that of the primary caregiver) presented simultaneously with music would have even greater benefits in alleviating physiological stress responses. Without substantial evidence from well-designed studies, however, it is difficult to draw such a conclusion. The effects of mother's voice have not been adequately studied beyond infancy; therefore, the responses of children to music combined with mother's voice are presently unknown. Additionally, the degree to which preferred music, or the combination of preferred music with mother's voice, would have a sedating effect on critically ill children has yet to be sufficiently researched. Last, when evaluating music to sedate and relax critically ill infants and children, important outcomes such as the decreased need for pharmacotherapy and length of stay in the CCU must be accurately and reliably measured.

SECONDARY TREATMENT GOALS

Secondary treatment goals for children in critical care may address general sensory stimulation, environmental awareness, or emotional coping issues. Children who are recovering from brain injury or disease of the brain, or have been extremely deconditioned due to cardiac, renal or respiratory issues progress medically to a point where attention to functional motoric, cognitive, and/or communication skills is needed in addition to calming and relaxation. For those patients with higher cognitive function who require long-term electronic monitoring of vital signs, drainage tubes, or mechanical supports, development of adapted meaningful leisure skills is indicated.

OUTCOME MEASURES

Outcome measures for treatment may be physiological, behavioral, psychosocial, or typically, a combination of all three. Physiological measures include heart rate, respiratory rate, blood pressure, requirements for sedation or analgesics, and oxygen saturation levels. Investigations across the medical literature support the use of music to produce favorable responses in these physiological outcomes, as well as galvanic skin responses, and electroencephalographic alpha brain waves (Standley, 2000). In a recent study of children with environmentally-induced autonomic dysfunction, music therapy presented twice daily for 20–30 minutes at fixed times for a duration of 3 weeks produced return of normotension (Sidorenko, 2000). Table 3 summarizes developmental guidelines for normal physiological ranges and target resting rates (Hazinski, 1992; Curley et al., 1996). While these guidelines provide general target ranges, optimum levels are individualized and variable depending on the type of medical condition, sedation, and/or vital supports involved. For those children on mechanical ventilation, breath rate and oxygen saturation levels are largely regulated by settings on the ventilator, and therefore do not vary widely as a response to stress or relaxation. Determination of appropriate treatment goals should be made in conjunction with the child's primary nurse or attending physician.

Table 3
Pediatric Vital Sign Parameters

	Neonate	Infant	1-2 yr	3-5 yr	6-9 yr
Heart Rate (bpm)	100–180	100–160	80–110	70–110	65–110
Respiratory Rate (pm)	30–60	30–60	25–35	20–30	18–30
Systolic Blood Pressure	60–90	88–105	95–105	90–110	95–115
Diastolic Blood Pressure	20–60	52–65	55–65	55–65	56–70

Note. Baseline normal range for patient should be correlated.

Behavioral outcomes include decreased crying, moaning, restlessness and agitated movement. For those children who are less sedated, increased quiet listening, visual attending, and passive interaction through assisted communication (i.e., yes/no responses, visual or tactile choice of songs and instruments) is appropriate.

Psychosocial outcomes for children who are less sedated involve calm interaction. Demonstration of neutral to bright affect is one indicator of coping in pediatric patients. For some children, indicators of affect may be determined more appropriately by expression through their eyes than through their mouths due to intubation, paralytic sedation, or injury to facial structure. Offering choices and assisting the child to communicate their preferences, when possible, transfers the locus of control to the patient and allows for measured self expression. Attention to family-centered care places importance on increased involvement of parents or significant caregivers, not only in determination of appropriate music, but through active participation in music play with or for the child. In this way, the child and the family may experience more familiar and normal interaction patterns in the midst of an anxiety producing situation.

REFERRAL, DOCUMENTATION, AND PRECAUTIONS

Best practice methods include the development of a referral process and routine methods of communication with the critical care physicians and nurses. Referrals may come through physician consult or an established protocol with nursing. Treatment goals and plans developed in conjunction with the child's primary nurse or attending physician will ensure appropriate outcome targets, cooperation with scheduling, and continuity of care and collection of data for evaluation. Routine progress notes kept in the patient chart communicate treatment procedures and progress to all healthcare professionals involved in the child's care.

Review of the chart and communication with nursing will also ensure that the music therapist remains in compliance with activity restrictions and possible infection control procedures. Physicians generally document the degree and type of movement and activity medically permitted, given the condition of the child. Proper donning of medical gowns, gloves, and masks by the music therapist may be needed to protect patients with weakened immune functions. Additionally, protection may need to be taken from specific infections or bacteria harbored in a patient's secretions. When indicated, isolation precautions are necessary to protect the patient, the therapist, and more typically, to prevent the spread of bacteria to other similarly vulnerable patients. Hospitals have established infection control procedures posted for review. Given the music therapist's interaction and use of instruments from patient to patient, a high level of routine infection control through use of germicidal wipes or spray must be maintained.

EXPERIMENTAL INVESTIGATION

One treatment model for critically ill children on mechanical ventilation is a protocol being developed at the Penn State Milton S. Hershey Medical Center in Hershey, Pennsylvania, based on a study funded in part by the Arthur Flagler Fultz Research Award of the American Music Therapy Association (Stouffer, Shirk, & Polomano, 2001). Approval for the research was applied for and granted by the Internal Review Board for Protection of Human Subjects within the hospital. This clinical investigation was designed by a collaborative team consisting of nursing researchers and music therapists in consultation with the Director of Pediatric Critical Care and the Department of Audiology. The intent was to document the impact of a specific music protocol as an adjunct to the routine clinical care of mechanically ventilated children.

Aims

The purpose of the study was to compare the effects of three audiotapes (a blank audiotape, music alone, and simultaneous music and mother's voice) on physiological variables and level of sedation, to evaluate between-group differences and within-subject variability over time, to determine the immediate and short-term benefits of music alone and music and mother's voice, and to establish interrater reliability and concurrent validity for a sedation measure designed by the ICU for critically ill infants and children.

Sample Characteristics

Thirty-four subjects, ranging in age from 3 months to 8 years, and their primary caregivers were recruited from within the 12-bed Pediatric Intensive Care Unit of the Children's Hospital within this regional medical facility. Figure 3 summarizes the criteria established to determine eligibility of children for this research protocol.

Methods and Procedures

A repeated measures cross-over design was used for the study, with all nurse raters blinded as to treatment condition. All subjects who passed a hearing screening were assigned to receive six audiotape trials, two each of a blank audiotape for control, music alone, and simultaneous music

Inclusion Criteria	*Exclusion Criteria*
• Age 3 month to 8 years	• Hemodynamically unstable or end of life
• Receiving mechanical ventilation	• Known or suspected active seizure disorder
• 24 hours after admission to the PICU	• Glascow Coma Scale < 5
• Primary caregiver willing to participate	• Evidence of hearing impairment
• Albuterol received by continuous infusion	

Figure 3. *Subject Eligibility Criteria*

and mother's (or primary caregiver's) voice. The three conditions were presented in random order, then repeated. Outcome measures consisted of heart rate (HR), respiratory rate (RR), blood pressure (BP), and oxygen saturation level (O_2 Sat). Sedation scores were recorded using both the Penn State Levels of Sedation Scale (Appendix B) and the Sedation-Agitation Scale (Riker et al., 1994) (Appendix A). In the absence of a validated tool for pediatric sedation, the latter adult-focused scale was determined to be appropriate for this study.

Once formal written consent was obtained by parents or guardians for participation of the child and themselves, all pediatric subjects were evaluated by an audiologist for hearing acuity. An auditory brainstem response (ABR) screening was administered and interpreted by certified audiologists to assess the patients' auditory function. The ABR was administered at a level of 35 dBnHL, which is the recommended screening level to ensure hearing that is adequate for speech recognition (AAA, 1999; Joint Committee on Infant Hearing, 1994; Stach & Santilli, 1998). When an ABR is present at this level, a moderate to profound hearing loss in the speech frequency region, including but not limited to 2000–4000 Hz, can be ruled out. Therefore, any child with a response at 35 dBnHL in at least one ear was included in the study. Results were often confounded by environmental noise and testing was repeated to confirm functionality. All results of the ABR screening were charted for the patient's attending physician who then discussed the outcome with parents if the screening failed.

Demographic information (e.g., age, gender, social history), medical diagnosis, medical history, date of admission to the PICU, date and time of mechanical ventilation, and treatments, procedures and medication profile were collected (Appendix C). The music therapist investigator interviewed the mother or primary caregiver to determine the music selections to be used for the audiotapes. Based on information highlighted in the interview, the caregiver chose songs that best incorporated the child's preference for music that was known to have a relaxing or calming effect on that child. Any known adverse effects of music were also discussed. A summary of the sample characteristics and demographic information with respect to music experiences and preferences are summarized in Appendix D. Initially, the field for selection of music was completely open ended. If caregivers had difficulty bringing specific music to mind, a list of possible selections was provided as a cue for recall and decision making. The list consisted of a wide categorical variety, including traditional children's songs suggested by the Humpal study (1998), classical pieces, lullabies, Bible songs and spirituals, and cultural selections reflective of the predominant demographics of the region served by this hospital. In addition to these categories, several

Table 4
Preferred Music for Research Audiotapes According to Frequency of Selection

Song Title	# of Times Requested
Jesus Loves Me	16
Twinkle, Twinkle Little Star	15
You Are My Sunshine	14
Barney Song (I Love You)	12
Itsy Bitsy Spider	9
Brahm's Lullaby	9
Rock-a-Bye Baby	9
Jesus Loves the Little Children	7
This Little Light of Mine	7
Somewhere Over the Rainbow	6
Winnie the Pooh	6
Hush Little Baby	5
All the Pretty Little Horses	4
Are You Sleeping	4
He's Got the Whole World	4
I've Been Workin' on the Railroad	4
London Bridge	3
Mary Had a Little Lamb	3
Angels Among Us	2
Arms Wide Open	2
Children's Prayer	2
I Love the Mountains	2
Kumbaya	2
Love Without End, Amen	2
Minuet in G	2
Skinnamerink-a-Dink	2
Sesame Street Theme Song	2
This Old Man (I Love You)	2
Whisper a Prayer	2
All Night All Day	1
Arabic Style Music	1
Candle on the Water	1
Circle of Life	1
De Colores	1
Down in the Valley	1
Hero	1
His Banner of Love	1
Lord Is My Shepherd, The	1
Oh Shenandoah	1
Old MacDonald	1
Sleep, Baby, Sleep	1
Whole New World, A	1
Peace Like a River	1
Deep and Wide	1
Father, We Thank Thee	1

families added country or pop tunes that were of a ballad nature. Upon completion of the study, a list of all music chosen for use on the audiotapes was compiled according to frequency of selection (see Table 4).

Within the patient's reported preference, appropriate music selections were chosen to create a 20-minute treatment condition. Individualized audiotapes were prepared for each child, adapting approximately 7 to 9 pieces of their preferred music to reflect accepted qualities of sedative music as outlined in the review of literature. Musical components of the recorded selections are summarized in Figure 4.

- Melody performed on electric piano
- Melodic line moving in step-wise increments with minimal interval jumps
- Arpeggiated chordal accompaniment played on classical guitar
- Mid-range tunes with avoidance of high frequencies
- Tempo of 60–72 bpm
- Smooth and consistent rhythm, without sudden changes
- Soft to moderately loud volume, approximately 65–70 dB

Figure 4. *Musical Components of Research Audiotapes*

For addition of the voice component to the music and voice condition, the therapist gave primary caregivers the option of singing along with the chosen selections or reading. Family could select a book either from their personal library or from resources provided. If the parent chose to sing, lyrics were provided. The therapist developed the 20-minute tapes using a Roland digital multitrack recorder. The music selection for each tape, both music alone and music paired with caregiver's voice, was the same, copied directly from the hard drive. The caregiver's voice was mixed onto the second tape by adding a track while listening to the recorded selections. By following the above guidelines for creating individualized recorded tapes, the team ensured consistency of musical quality and presentation across subjects even though specific content selection varied according to preference.

The audiotapes were played using a Sony Walkman WM-FX251 and presented to subjects through Sony MDR-CD 160 stereo headphones that provided total ear coverage. These headphones consisted of a plastic head strap and vinyl-covered ear pads that could be wiped with germicidal cleaner after use on each child. Presentation level of the audiotapes was preset by the audiologist at 70 dBSPL. This level was chosen for two reasons. First, speech frequencies range in intensity from 40–70 dBSPL (Skinner, 1978). Secondly, the ambient noise levels measured in the hospital's PICU with a dosimeter averaged 67.6 dBSPL. A presentation level of 70 dBSPL ensured that all frequencies were audible, and that the output of the cassette player was above the intensity of the ambient noise. To enhance the attenuation of the ambient noise, the Sony headphones were used. A sound level meter was used to calibrate the output of the audio cassette players. A 1 kHz pure tone recorded on a standard cassette tape was used to set the output to 70 dBSPL using an A-weighted scale (Cudahy, 1988). Following this calibration, the volume control was secured to maintain a consistent volume level within and across subjects for all trials.

Nurse data collectors were trained as to study procedures and data collection methods. Research materials, including a box of treatment tapes that were identified by color code only, a precleaned tape player and headset, a data collection notebook, and extra batteries were given to each subject's nurse. Attempts were made to obtain two trials per 8-hour shift; however due to a variety of conditions, actual timing was inconsistent. Within the context of routine medical care, the subject's nurse determined an appropriate time during his or her 8-hour shift when the child exhibited signs of agitation. Figure 5 summarizes the protocol used by nurses involved in the study to determination appropriate timing for initiation of the research audiotapes.

- Penn State Level of Sedation ranging between 2 and 4
- Minimum of 1 hour since last intermittent dose of sedation/analgesic
- 2 or more hours since end of previous MT audiotape trial

Figure 5. *Nursing Protocol for Initiation of Research Audiotapes*

For each trial, the nurse selected the appropriate color coded tape and applied the headset with earphones placed securely over the infant's or child's ears. The headset was placed on the subject before initiation of the audiotape to prevent the possibility of trial contents being heard by the nurse. Following a baseline recording of all physiological and sedation level assessments, the tape player was turned to the on position. Measures were then documented at 5, 10, and 20 minutes following initiation of the tape. The tape ended after 20 minutes. Two additional assessments were taken at 30 and 60 minutes after the start of the tape, then headsets were removed. If at any time during the trial the child exhibited increased signs of agitation or worsening of physiological parameters, additional medications were available for administration. Dosages of intermittent analgesics and sedating agents were recorded during the study.

If parents or caregivers were present during the audiotape trials, they were instructed not to speak to or touch the child for the 60-minute data collection period. This was requested to control for any effects that interaction may have had on the child, and agreed on during the formal consent process. Between trials, research materials were kept by the bedside, then collected upon completion of the final trial. Subjects were required to have completed a data set of at least three of the six trials, one of each condition, for inclusion with statistical analysis. Repeated measure analysis of variance (ANOVA) was used to determine within-subject and treatment differences over time for physiological variables and level of sedation.

Results

Detailed analysis of statistical results is currently being submitted for publication. In summary, subjects were significantly more sedated while listening to music and mother's voice at 15 and 20 minutes after the audiotape was initiated. Overall mean systolic blood pressure was significantly lower for trials with music alone (MA) and music and mother's voice (MMV) compared to the blank audiotape (BA) trials. No significant treatment effects were evident for heart rate or respiratory rate. Overall mean O_2 saturation level was statistically lower for MMV from BA and MA; however, this decrease was not clinically meaningful and may have resulted from greater sedation and decreased spontaneous minute volume. No measurable carry-over effects were observed on physiological outcomes once audiotapes were discontinued.

Conclusions

Based upon the results of this pilot study, music combined with mother's voice appeared to be more effective than music alone or the control tape of silence in maintaining desired levels of sedation with children on mechanical ventilation. Additional analysis is needed to correlate exact dosages of sedation and analgesic required by the subjects during the various time intervals of the study. Music and mother's voice was associated with a reduction in systolic blood pressure during the interval when the audiotape was played compared to music alone and the blank audiotape.

Greater numbers of subjects are needed to establish statistically significant and clinically meaningful differences on physiological variables. Given the medical parameters for maintaining stability of vital signs in the PCCU, treatment effect for the use of therapeutic music in this setting is likely to be relatively small. Therefore a greater sample size is needed for power of analysis. Most parents were agreeable to having their child participate in the study. Of those parents who declined consent, the majority responded in a manner that indicated a tendency to be overwhelmed with the critical care experience and a withdrawal from needing to make another decision regarding the care of their child. Future investigations will need to account for increased stress levels when approaching parents or guardians for consent.

Particular attention should be paid to development of criteria regarding determination of need for intermittent sedating agents during the course of the study. Pediatric patients are prescribed a desired level of sedation and baseline dosages of sedative medication. Upon signs of increased patient agitation, nurses routinely administer bolus dosages as needed to maintain the sedation level. Investigators of this study noted reluctance on the part of the subjects' primary nurses to attempt initiation of treatment trials when agitation was first observed. Bolus dosages were often administered at a frequency which precluded initiation of audiotape trials. These observations are supported by a survey of critical care nurses caring for adult patients receiving mechanical ventilation (Weinert, Chlan, & Gross, 2001). Nurses interviewed identified the following goals for sedation: to increase the comfort of their patients, to induce amnesia so patients will not remember the critical care experience, and to prevent self-injurious behavior. Nurses readily acknowledged that other factors, including influence by family members, time constraints, and communication with physicians, affected their practice as well. In general, development of valid measurement of sedation efficacy remains an important issue among critical care providers (Hansen-Flaschen, Cowen, & Polomano, 1994). Additional education as to potential effects of music treatment conditions and an algorithm for subsequently administering sedatives and analgesic is highly recommended.

Finally, therapeutic music may not lead to significant decreases in heart rate with critically ill children due to numerous confounding pathophysiological variables and regulatory medications. Anecdotal observations of several subjects noted by nurse recorders pointed to a trend for increased calm listening and decreased agitated movement during trials that were conducted when subjects were experiencing a higher level of awareness.

Discussion

This pilot study was successful in establishing the groundwork for future research in the application of music with critically ill children on mechanical ventilation. Through collaborative teamwork by nurses, music therapists, trained researchers, audiologists, and the Director of Pediatric Critical Care, a detailed methodological design was established that met criteria for scientific rigor and followed principles published to date on the use of developmentally appropriate music for relaxation and sedation. Clinically meaningful procedures were developed and approved for conducting the research within the context of routine medical care, meeting regulatory standards for critical care, safety and infection control, and patient confidentiality. Future efforts will need to examine outcome variables and determine more appropriate means of measuring treatment effect with this population. While physiological outcomes consisting of routine vital signs yield clinically and statistically meaningful results when observed in other populations, medical management of critically ill children precludes variability of these physiological indicators. Consideration may be given to outcomes and target variables under study within the body of psychoneuroimmunological (PNI) research. Additional directions may include use of emerging medical technology such as the Bispectral Index (BIS) monitor which quantifies achieved levels of sedation by means of a processed cortical electroencephalogram (EEG) (Denman et al., 2000).

CLINICAL PROTOCOL

Based on the previously described pilot study, a clinical protocol was developed and approved by the Critical Care Committee for routine use at the investigator's medical facility (see Figure 6). A data base of adapted preferred music considered to be calming to children age 3 months to 8 years was created. Songs were categorized according to musical style, sacred versus secular content, and developmental level. Each category was recorded on CD and timed for 20 minutes of playing. These musically adapted, individualized CD collections will be kept on the critical care unit, along with CD players and headphones, for nurses to use as an immediate compliment to sedation. Parents or primary caregivers will select the CD or CDs they consider to be most appropriate for their child, and educated as to procedures and schedule for playing. Parents of those children who will remain on the ventilator for more than 48 hours will be interviewed personally by the music therapist and given the option to individualize the music selections further, and to add their voice as a track on the CD. Outcome measures and method of selection and presentation of music will continue to be refined.

It is anticipated that through use and refinement of this protocol with children on mechanical ventilation, procedures may be developed for generalization of use with other critically ill children receiving high levels of sedation or experiencing low levels of awareness.

CONCLUSION

Music therapists play a vital role in determining the extent to which music will become a routine, complimentary treatment in the pediatric critical care setting. While awareness of treatment applications among healthcare professionals has increased, the need for education and

Target Population

- Children 3 months through 8 years admitted to the PICU
- Mechanical ventilation
- Sedation required to achieve Penn State Level Of Sedation (PSLOS) 2-4
- No history of hearing loss
- No active or suspected seizure disorder

Protocol

First 24 hours of admission:

1. On admission to the PICU, staff will explain use of Music Therapy (MT) to parents.
2. Staff/parents will select CD from supply available in the unit. Other selections to accommodate individualized spiritual/cultural needs are available through MT staff.
3. When patient is showing signs of wakefulness/agitation, the RN will apply the headphones and start the CD. If the child continues to show signs of agitation beyond desired PSLOS, the RN will administer sedatives as needed.
4. CDs should be offered during resting periods to encourage sedation and rest. CDs will not be initiated during invasive procedures (ie: suctioning), but immediately following for calming. No more than two applications will be given in any 3 hour period. 15+ minute breaks between CDs is suggested.

Following 48 hours (if continued intubation expected):

1. Family will be offered opportunity to record and mix their voice with music.
2. MT will be paged for scheduling interview and recording.
3. When patient is showing signs of wakefulness/agitation, the RN will apply the headphones and start the CD. If the child continues to show signs of agitation beyond desired PSLOS, the RN will administer sedatives as needed.
4. CDs should be offered during resting periods to encourage sedation and rest. CDs will not be initiated during invasive procedures (ie: suctioning), but immediately following for calming. No more than two applications will be given in any 3 hour period. 15+ minute breaks between CDs is suggested.

Following Extubation:

1. Clean and return headphones and CD player to bin located on the unit
2. Return general CDs to bin located in the unit
3. Give CDs individualized with parent voice to family.

Figure 6. *Clinical Protocol for Use of Music with Critically Ill Children on Mechanical Ventilation*

development of reliable treatment protocols remains. Investigative progress is being made; however, methodologically sound research conducted by teams that include both music therapists and healthcare professionals is still needed to answer important questions regarding selection and presentation of music, duration and frequency of treatments, and appropriate methods of evaluation. Treatment protocols for specific ages and populations that can be validated, replicated and incorporated into care will provide a standardized basis for addressing the biomedical and psychosocial needs of critically ill children and their families. The crucial task will be to achieve these standards while maintaining the unique individuality of the relationship between music, patient and therapist.

Support for research to develop this treatment protocol was granted by the Arthur Flagler Fultz Research Fund of the American Music Therapy Association.

REFERENCES

American Academy of Audiology (AAA). (1999). *Position statement.* Available: http://www.audiology.org

Bailey, L. (1983). The effects of live music versus tape-recorded music on hospitalized cancer patients. *Music Therapy, 3*(1), 17–28.

Barrera, M., Rykov, M., & Doyle, S. (2002). The effects of interactive music therapy on hospitalized children with cancer: A pilot study. *Psycho-Oncology, 11*, 379–388.

Berlin, B. (1998). Music therapy with children during invasive procedures: Our emergency department's experience. *Journal of Emergency Nursing, 24*(6), 607–608.

Bonny, H. (1983). Music listening for intensive coronary care units: a pilot project. *Music Therapy, 3*(1), 4–16.

Bonny, H. (1986). Music and healing. *Music Therapy, 6A*(1), 3–12.

Brackbill, Y., Adams, G., Crowell, D., & Gray, M. (1966). Arousal level in neonates and preschool children under continuous auditory stimulation. *Journal of Experimental Child Psychology, 4*, 178–188.

Brattebo, G., Hofoss, D., Flatten, H., & Muri, A. K., Gjerde, S., & Plsek, P. E. (2002). Effect of a scoring system and protocol for sedation on duration of patients' need for ventilator support in a surgical intensive care unit. *British Medical Journal, 324*(7350), 1386–1389.

Burke, M., Walsh, J., Oehler, J., & Gingras, J. (1995). Music therapy following suctioning: Four case studies. *Neonatal Network, 14*(7), 41–49.

Byers, J. F., & Smyth, K. A. (1997). Effect of a music intervention on noise annoyance, heart rate, and blood pressure in cardiac surgery patients. *American Journal of Critical Care, 6*(3), 183–191.

Cabrera, I., & Lee, H. (2000). Reducing noise pollution in the hospital setting by establishing a department of sound: A survey of recent research on the effects of noise and music in health care. *Preventive Medicine, 30*, 339–345.

Caine, J. (1991). The effects of music on the selected stress behaviors, weight, caloric and formula intake, and length of hospital stay for premature and low birth weight neonates in a newborn intensive care unit. *Journal of Music Therapy, 28*(4), 180–192.

Caire, J., & Erickson, S. (1986). Reducing distress in pediatric patients undergoing cardiac catheterization. *Children's Health Care, 14*(3), 146–152.

Cassidy, J., & Ditty, K. (1998). Presentation of aural stimuli to newborns and premature Infants: an audiological perspective. *Journal of Music Therapy, 35*(2), 70–87.

Cassidy, J., & Standley, J. (1995). The effect of music listening on physiological responses of premature infants in the NICU. *Journal of Music Therapy, 32(4*), 180–192.

Chetta, H. (1981). The effect of music and desensitization on preoperative anxiety in children. *Journal of Music Therapy, 18*, 74–87.

Chlan, L. (1998). Effectiveness of a music therapy intervention on relaxation and anxiety for patients receiving ventilatory assistance. *Heart and Lung, 27*(3), 169–176.

Chlan, L. (2000). Music therapy as a nursing intervention for patients supported by mechanical ventilation. *AACN Clinical Issues, 11*(1), 128–138.

Chlan, L., & Tracy, M. (1999). Music therapy in critical care: Indications and guidelines for intervention. *Critical Care Nurse, 19*(3), 35–41.

Christenberry, E. (1979). The use of music therapy with burn patients. *Journal of Music Therapy, 16*, 138–148.

Cudahy, E. (1988). *Introduction to instrumentation in speech and hearing.* Baltimore: Williams & Wilkens.

Curley, M., Smith, J., & Moloney-Harmon, P. (1996). *Critical care nursing of infants and children.* Philadelphia: W. B. Saunders.

Davis, W., Gfeller, K., & Thaut, M. (1992). *An introduction to music therapy theory and practice*. Dubuque, IA: Wm. C. Brown.

Davis, W., & Thaut, M. (1989). The influence of preferred relaxing music on measures of state anxiety, relaxation, and physiological responses. *Journal of Music Therapy, 26*(4), 168–187.

Dengerink, H., Wright, J., Thompson, P., & Dengerink, J. (1982). Changes in plasma angiotensin II with noise exposure and their relationship to TTS. *Journal of the Acoustical Society of America, 72*, 276–278.

Denman, W., Swanson, E., Rosow, D., Ezbicki, K., Connors, P., & Rosow, C. (2000). Pediatric evaluation of the bispectral index (BIS) monitor and correlation of BIS with end-tidal sevoflurane concentration in infants and children. *Anesthesia & Analgesia, 90*(4), 872–877.

Dun, B. (1995). A different beat: Music therapy in children's cardiac care. *Music Therapy Perspectives, 13*, 35–39.

Fontaine, D. (1994). Nonpharmacologic management of patient distress during mechanical ventilation. *Critical Care Clinics, 10*(4), 695–708.

Fowler-Kerry, S., & Lander, J. (1987). Management of injection pain in children. *Pain, 30*, 169–175.

Gaston, E. (1968). Man and music. In E. Gaston (Ed.), *Music in therapy* (pp. 7–29). New York: Macmillan.

Grasso, M., Button, M., Allison, D., & Sawyer, S. (2000). Benefits of music therapy as an adjunct to chest physiotherapy in infants and toddlers with cystic fibrosis. *Pediatric Pulmonology, 29*, 371–381.

Guzzetta, C. (1995). Music therapy: Hearing the melody of the soul. In B. Dossey, L. Keegan, C. Guzzetta, & L. Kolkmeier, (Eds.), *Holistic nursing* (pp. 669–698). Gaithersburg, MD: Aspen.

Hansen-Flaschen, J., Cowen, J., & Polomano, R. (1994). Beyond the Ramsay scale: Need for a validated measure of sedating drug efficacy in the intensive care unit. *Critical Care Medicine,*

22(5), 732–733.

Hazinski, M. F. (Ed.). (1992). Nursing care of the critically ill child (2nd ed). Salem, MA: Mosby-Year Book.

Heitz, L., Symreng, T., & Scamman, F. (1992). The use of music during the immediate postanesthesia care unit: A nursing intervention. *Journal of Post Anesthesia Nursing, 7*(1), 22–31.

Humpal, M. (1998). Song repertoire of young children. *Music Therapy Perspectives, 16*(1), 37–42.

Joint Committee on Infant Hearing (JCIH). (1994). Joint Committee on Infant Hearing: 1994 position statement. *ASHA, 33,* 3–6.

Kagan, J., & Lewis, M. (1965). Studies of attention in the human infant. *Merrill-Palmer Quarterly, 11,* 95–127.

Kallay, V. (1997). Music therapy applications in the pediatric medical setting: Child development, pain management and choices. In J. Loewy (Ed.), *Music therapy and pediatric pain* (pp. 33–43). Cherry Hill, NJ: Jeffrey Books.

Keller, V. (1995). Management of nausea and vomiting in children. *Journal of Pediatric Nursing, 10*(5), 280–286.

Klein, S., & Winkelstein, M. (1996). Enhancing pediatric health care with music. *Journal of Pediatric Health Care, 10,* 74–81.

Koch, M., Kain, Z., Ayoub, C., & Rosenbaum, S. (1998). The sedative and analgesic sparing effect of music. *Anesthesiology, 89*(2), 300–306.

Lepage, C., Drolet, P., Girard, M., Grenier, Y., & DeGagne, R. (2001). Music decreases sedative requirements during spinal anesthesia. *Anesthesia and Analgesia, 93,* 912–916.

Lewandowski, L. (1992). Psychosocial aspects of pediatric critical care. In M. Hazinski (Ed.), *Nursing care of the critically ill child* (pp. 19–77). St. Louis, MO: Mosby Year Book.

Loewy, J., MacGregor, B., Richards, K., & Rodriquez, J. (1997). Music therapy pediatric pain management: Assessing and attending to the sounds of hurt, fear, and anxiety. In J. Loewy (Ed.), *Music therapy and pediatric pain* (pp. 45–55). Cherry Hill, NJ: Jeffrey Books.

Lovallo, W., & Pishkin, V. (1980). A psycho physiological comparison of type A and B men exposed to failure and uncontrollable noise. *Psychophysiology, 17*(1), 29–36.

Malone, A. (1996). The effects of live music on the distress of pediatric patients receiving intravenous starts, venipunctures, injections, and heel sticks. *Journal of Music Therapy, 33*(1), 19–33.

McLean, I., & Tarnopolsky, A. (1977). Noise discomfort and mental health. *Psychological Medicine, 7,* 19–62.

Micci, N. (1984). The use of music therapy with pediatric patients undergoing cardiac catheterization. *The Arts in Psychotherapy, 11,* 261–266.

Monroe, J. (1996). How noise pollution affects us. *Current Health 2, 22*(7), 30–32.

Nilsson, U., Rawal, N., Unestahl, L., Zetterberg, C., & Unosson, M. (2001). Improved recovery after music and therapeutic suggestions during general anaesthesia: A double-blind randomized controlled trial. *Acta Anaesthesiol Scand, 45,* 812–817.

Ochiai, N., Okutani, R., Yoshimura, Y., & Fu, K. (1995). Perioperative management of a patient with severe bronchial asthma attack. *Masui, 44*(8), 1124–1127.

Pfaff, V., Smith, K., & Gowan, D. (1989). The effects of music-assisted relaxation on the distress on pediatric cancer patients undergoing bone marrow aspirations. *Children's Health Care, 18*(4), 232–236.

Rasco, C. (1992). Using music therapy as distraction during lumbar punctures. *Journal of Pediatric Oncology Nursing, 9*(1), 33–34.

Rider, M. (1997). *The rhythmic language of health and disease*. St. Louis, MO: MMB Music.

Riker, R., Fraser, G., & Cox, P. (1994). Continuous infusion of haloperidol controls agitation in critically ill patients. *Critical Care Medicine, 22*(3), 433–440.

Robb, S., Nichols, R., Rutan, R., Bishop, B., & Parker, J. (1995). The effects of music assisted relaxation on perioperative anxiety. *Journal of Music Therapy, 32*(1), 2–21.

Robb, S.(2000). The effect of therapeutic music interventions on the behavior of hospitalized children in isolation: Developing a contextual support model of music therapy. *Journal of Music Therapy, 37*(2), 118–146.

Rosenfeld, J., & Dun, B. (1999). Music therapy in children with severe traumatic brain injury. In R. R. Pratt & D. E. Grocke (Eds.), *Music medicine 3* (pp. 35–46). Victoria, Australia: The University of Melbourne.

Scartelli, J. (1989). *Music and self-management methods: A physiological model* (pp. 20–24). St. Louis MO: MMB Music.

Sidorenko, V. (2000). Effects of the medical resonance therapy music on haemodynamic parameter in children with autonomic nervous system disturbances. *Integrative Physiological and Behavioral Science, 35*(3), 208–211.

Skinner, M. (1978). The hearing of speech during language acquisition. *Otolaryngological Clinics of North America, 11,* 631–50.

Spintge, R. (1989). The anxiolytic effects of music. In M. Lee (Ed.), *Rehabilitation, music and human well-being* (pp. 82–97). St. Louis, MO: MMB Music.

Stach, B., & Santilli, C. (1998). Technology in newborn hearing screening. In S. H. Morgan (Ed.), *Universal newborn hearing screening: seminars in hearing, 19*(3), 247–261.

Stanley, J. (2000). Music research in medical treatment. In *Effectiveness of music therapy procedures: Documentation of research and clinical practice* (3rd ed., pp. 1–64). Silver Spring, MD: American Music Therapy Association.

Standley, J. (2002). A meta-analysis of the efficacy of music therapy for premature infants. *Journal of Pediatric Nursing, 17*(2), 107–113.

Standley, J., & Madsen, C. (1990). Comparison of infant preferences and responses to auditory stimuli: Music, mother, and other female voice. *Journal of Music Therapy, 27*(2), 54–97.

Standley, J., & Moore, R. (1995). Therapeutic effects of music and mother's voice on premature infants. *Pediatric Nursing, 21*(6), 509–512.

Steinke, W. (1991). The use of music, relaxation, and imagery in the management of postsurgical pain for scoliosis. In C. Maranto (Ed.), *Applications of music in medicine* (pp. 141–162). Washington, DC: National Association for Music Therapy.

Stouffer, J., Shirk, B., & Polomano, R. (2001). *A comparison of music to music with mother's voice on physiological responses and level of sedation with critically ill infants and children.* Paper presented at 2001 American Music Therapy Association Conference, Pasadena, CA.

Tang, C., Ko, C. J., Ng, S., Chen, S., Cheng, K., Yu, K., & Tseng, C. (1993). "Walkman music" during epidural anesthesia. *Kao Hsiung I Hsuch Ko Hsueh Tsa Chich, 9*(8), 468–475.

Tryba, M. (1996). Choices in sedation: The balanced sedation technique. *European Journal of Anaesthesiology Supplement, 13*, 8–12.

Weinert, C., Chlan, L., & Gross, C. (2001). Sedating critically ill patients: Factors affecting nurses' delivery of sedative therapy. *American Journal of Critical Care, 10*(3), 156–167.

Whipple, J. (2000). The effect of parent training in music and multimodal stimulation on parent-neonate interactions in the neonatal intensive care unit. *Journal of Music Therapy, 37*(4), 250–268.

Wong, H., Lopez-Nahas, V., & Molassiotis, A. (2001). Effects of music therapy on anxiety in ventilator-dependent patients. *Heart & Lung, 30*(5), 376–387.

Zifkin, B., & Andermann, F. (2001). Epilepsy with reflex seizures. In E. Wyllie (Ed.), *The treatment of epilepsy: Principles and practice* (pp. 537–649). Philadelphia: Lippincott, Williams & Wilkins.

APPENDIX A

Sedation-Agitation Scale

7	Dangerous agitation	Pulling at endotracheal tube, trying to remove catheters, climbing over bed rail, striking at staff, thrashing side to side.
6	Very agitated	Does not calm, despite frequent verbal reminding of limits; requires physical restraints, biting endotracheal tube.
5	Agitated	Anxious or mildly agitated, attempting to sit up, calms down to verbal instructions.
4	Calm and cooperative	Calm, awakens easily, follows commands.
3	Sedated	Difficult to arouse, awakens to verbal stimuli or gentle shaking but drifts off again, follows simple commands.
2	Very sedated	Arouses to physical stimuli but does not communicate or follow commands, may move spontaneously.
1	Unarousable	Minimal or no response to noxious stimuli, does not communicate or follow commands.

Riker, R. R., Picard, J. T., & Fraser, G. L. (1999). Prospective evaluation of the Sedation-Agitation Scale for adult critically ill patients. *Critical Care Medicine, 27*(7),1325–1329.

APPENDIX B

PennState Children's Hospital
Levels of Sedation Scale

Pediatric Intensive/Intermediate Care Unit
Levels of Sedation for Ventilated Patients

Level 1: Awake and **interactive** with environment, watches TV, communicates (generally for more mature children with neuromuscular cause for ventilation).
PRN sedatives.

Level 2: Sleepy, **arouses to light stimulation,** becomes excited with nursing care/ suctioning, moves spontaneously, turns head, consistently breathes above ventilator.
PRN sedatives, paralysis only for extreme agitation/movement

Level 3: Asleep most of the time, **arouses to pain,** coughs with suctioning, breathes above ventilator, **little spontaneous movement or head turning.**
PRN sedative, paralysis only if PRN sedatives fail

Level 4: Asleep, arouses to pain, coughs with suctioning**, returns to sleep immediately, does not consistently breathe above ventilator,** little spontaneous movement, no head turning.
PRN sedative, paralysis only if PRN sedatives fail

Level 5: Asleep, minimal response to pain or suctioning, **no respiratory effort, no spontaneous movements.**
PRN sedatives, liberal use of paralysis if PRN sedatives fail

Level 6: Asleep, **continuous paralysis,** level of paralysis assessed by nerve stimulator or by observing minor motor movements between supplemental doses.
PRN sedatives titrated to vital signs

 Revised 10/03/96

APPENDIX C

Demographic Data Sheet

Patient Name:________________________________ Date:________________

Date of Birth: ____________ Patient Number: ____________

Diagnosis: ______________________________ Weight: ___________

PICU Admission Date: ______________ Projected length of stay: ____________

Parent(s)/Guardian: ____

Telephone: (H)______________ (W)______________ (C) ________________

Address:____

____

Patient History

Is this your child's 1st hospitalization? _____YES _____NO

If no, how many times has he/she been hospitalized previously? __________

Is your child involved in any of the following? (check all that apply)

_____Day Care _____Toddler groups _____Pre-school

_____Kindergarten _____Elementary _____Grade _____Other____________

Optional statement of religious preference: ______________________________

Has your child had any exposure to music in groups, lessons, through family experiences?

_____YES _____NO If yes, please describe______________________________

Do you or a family member regularly sing to or around your child? _____YES _____NO

If yes, please list name and relationship to patient. ______________________

Has your child had any exposure to specific instruments? _____YES _____NO

If yes, please list: ____

Demographic Data **page 2**

Is music used as part of a regular routine for your child at any of the following times:

_____wake-up _____bath-time _____bed-time

_____getting dressed/morning routine _____other_____________________________

If any of the above are checked, please list what music and how it is used or presented to the child._____

To what music has your child been exposed in the home? (please check all that apply)

_____Children's songs _____Pop/rock _____Christian rock
_____Lullabies _____Folk _____Religious music
_____Holiday _____Jazz _____Traditional hymns
_____Classical _____New Age _____Bible songs
_____Cultural _____R&B _____Gospel
_____Country _____Other_____________________________

Does your child have a favorite song(s) or type of music? (please list) ____________________________

____

What music has been most calming to your child? (please list) ____________________________

____

Does your child have a favorite book(s)? (please list)____________________________

Has your infant or child reacted negatively (e.g., crying, agitation, restlessness, withdrawal, being upset) to any music experiences? _____YES _____NO

If yes, please describe:____________________________

Audiotape Preparation

For this study, would you or another primary caregiver like to _____SING or _____READ to your child?
Name of person providing voice: ____________________________

Preferred Selections:

APPENDIX D

Sample Characteristics		
Outcomes	**Mean**	***SD***
Age	1.61	1.61
Age Variables	*N*	**Percentage**
Age (*N* = 29)		
3–6 Months	6	20.70
7–9 Months	7	24.10
10–12Months	2	6.90
13–24 Months	6	20.70
25–36 Months (Year Two)	4	13.80
37–48 Months (Year Three)	1	3.50
49–60 Months (Year Four)	1	3.40
61–72 Months (Year Five)	1	3.50
87 Months (Year Seven)	1	3.40
Demographic Data		*N*
Diagnosis (*N* = 25)		
Respiratory Distress/Failure		9
Shunt Infection		1
Cardiomyopathy		1
Premature		1
Acute Liver Failure		1
Stab Wound		1
Heart Transplant		1
Hepatitis		1
Supraventricular Tachycardia		1
Spinal Muscular Atrophy		1
3rd Degree Burns		1
Leukemia		1
Kidney Disease		1
Subglottic Stenosis		1
TBI (Multiple Trauma)		1
Thrombosed Shunt		1
Pneumococcal Septic Shock		1

Demographic Data		*N*
Number of Hospitalizations ($N = 24$)		
First Time		9
One or More		15
# of Times = 1		9
# of Times = 2		8
# of Times = 3		1
# of Times = >3		6
Group Involvement ($N = 20$)		
Day Care		3
Toddler Group		2
Pre-School		4
Kindergarten		1
Elementary School		1
Other		6
None		3
Religious Preference ($N = 25$)		
Methodist		4
Pentecostal		1
Church of the Living God		2
Catholic		1
Moravian		1
Lutheran		1
Not Listed		15
Exposed to Music ($N = 25$)		
Yes		19
No		6
Where Was Child Exposed to Music		
Home		14
Church		3
Daycare		1
School		1
Other		3
Does Family Sing to Child? ($N = 21$)		
Yes		19
No		2

Demographic Data		*N*
Who Sings to Child? (*N* = 22)		9
Mother		2
Father		5
Both		6
Other		
Exposed to Specific Instruments? (*N* = 19)		
Yes		6
No		13
Type of Instrument		
Drums		1
Keyboard		2
Harmonica		2
Guitar		1
Other		1
Music Used as Part of Routines		
Wake-Up		1
Dressing/a.m.		0
Bath Time		2
Bed Time		8
Other		7
Caregiver Preference		
Sing		9
Read		12
No		2
Not Listed		6
Caregiver in Recording (*N* = 28)		
Mother		18
Father		6
Grandparent		1
Sibling		1
Other		2

FIVE

Neurologic Music Therapy With Children: Scientific Foundations and Clinical Application

Corene Hurt-Thaut, M.M., MT-BC
Sarah Johnson, M.M., MT-BC

FOR MANY YEARS, music therapists have demonstrated therapeutic success in using music for clinical applications with children. However, the lack of accountability and consistency in the use of music in therapy has made it impossible to reproduce consistent results, and has made goal-oriented, functional therapeutic application of music difficult. The result is that rational and effective therapeutic applications of music are often missed, ignored, or misapplied due to lack of understanding of the basic mechanisms involved in the perception and performance of music. Thaut (2000) proposed that in order to rationally translate musical experiences into therapeutic experiences, the following question needs to first be answered: What is the mechanism through which music psychologically and physiologically influences human behavior in a therapeutically meaningful and predictable way?

Music therapists have often tried to answer this question by doing outcome research to validate and quantify music therapy. This type of research, however, does not tell us how to translate music into therapy, which is the prerequisite for good music therapy research and clinical practice. The future growth of scientific and medical acceptance of music therapy depends on the development of models that can (a) explain the therapeutic effect of music on behavior based on scientific evidence, (b) provide the framework to systematically and creatively transform a musical response into a therapeutic response, and (c) develop a systematic clinical methodology to select applications and predict the therapeutic outcome and benefits (Thaut, 2000).

DEFINITION OF NEUROLOGIC MUSIC THERAPY

Neurologic Music Therapy (NMT) is defined as the therapeutic application of music to cognitive, sensory, and motor dysfunctions due to neurologic disease of the human nervous system. NMT is a research-based system of standardized clinical techniques for sensorimotor training, speech and language training, and cognitive training. NMT is used in neurologic rehabilitation, neuropediatric therapy, neurogeriatric therapy, and neurodevelopmental therapy. It is based on the *Rational Scientific Mediating Model (R-SMM),* a neuroscience model of music perception and production and the influence of music on functional changes in nonmusical brain and behavior function. Treatment techniques in NMT are based on scientific research, and are applied as *Therapeutic Music Interventions (TMI)*, which are adaptable to patient needs and functional therapeutic goals.

Clinical development and research efforts for Neurologic Music Therapy are coordinated through the Robert F. Unkefer Academy for Neurologic Music Therapy. In order to practice NMT, clinicians must receive specialized training in the theory and practice of NMT techniques through the academy. In addition to extensive training in NMT techniques, therapists practicing Neurologic Music Therapy are educated in the areas of neuroanatomy/physiology, brain pathologies, medical terminology, and rehabilitation of cognitive and motor functions (Thaut, Kenyon, Schauer, & McIntosh, 1999).

RATIONAL SCIENTIFIC MEDIATING MODEL

The Rational Scientific Mediating Model (R-SMM) is a model that explores the premise that the scientific basis of music therapy is found in the neurological, physiological, and psychological foundations of music perception and music production. It is essential to know how systems perceive, respond, and relate to music in order to build a meaningful connection between musical and non-musical behaviors. Only then, can music be translated into consistent therapeutic applications. The R-SMM is composed of four steps, which are all necessary in order to develop a valid model of music in therapy that will consistently modify behaviors in the cognitive, affective, and sensorimotor domains:

1. Musical Response Models: neurological, physiological, and psychological foundations of musical behavior;
2. Nonmusical Parallel Models: processes in nonmusical brain and behavior function;
3. Mediating Models: influence of music on nonmusical brain and behavior function;
4. Clinical Research Models: therapeutic effects of music.

Step 1: Musical Response Models

Step 1 in the R-SMM involves understanding music as an aesthetic object in which psychological and physiological responses are elicited through the perception and performance of musical stimuli. Berlyne (1971) identified the central nervous system as an arousal seeking system which seeks aesthetic input in order to satisfy the senses. Since music is an aesthetic object, it can be used as a mediator in the therapeutic process as a supplementary response which simulates a desired response in areas of cognition, affect, and motor performance. Psychological, collative, and ecological properties of music stimuli provide a structure which helps focus attention, increase motivation, and excite the senses, therefore meeting arousal needs.

Step 2: Nonmusical Parallel Models

Step 2 in the R-SMM involves identifying processes in nonmusical brain and behavior function and investigating whether there are similar processes involved in musical and nonmusical perception and behaviors which are of therapeutic interest. The question that needs to be answered in this step is whether there are parallels between affective, cognitive, and sensorimotor processes in musical and nonmusical behavior and perception.

Step 3: Mediating Models

Step 3 involves the development of mediating models based on the similarities and parallels identified in Step 2 in the affective, cognitive, and sensorimotor domains. The goal of these mediating models is to provide good theory and rationales for building future research hypotheses in order to be able to subsequently study the therapeutically meaningful influence of music on behavior and brain function (Thaut, 2000).

Step 4: Clinical Research Models

The last step of the R-SMM explores whether there is research evidence that supports the use of music with clinical populations. Through good clinical research, solid clinical techniques can be developed, therefore producing consistent outcomes when used in therapy.

Over the past 25 years, basic science and clinical research have answered many of the questions in all of the steps of the R-SMM related to the use of therapeutic music applications for sensorimotor, speech and communication, cognitive, and socioemotional rehabilitation.

STANDARDS OF BEST PRACTICE

According to the standards of best possible practice, treatment should be selected according to: (a) best available objective assessment procedures, and (b) best available objective outcome data. It only makes sense that patients deserve the best available treatment, and that it is the music therapist's responsibility to remain knowledgeable on what that is.

The R-SMM is a model that provides scientific evidence which explains the therapeutic effects of music on behavior, providing a framework for the systematic and creative transformation of musical responses into therapeutic responses that produce consistent therapeutic outcomes and benefits. Based on the evidence provided in the areas of cognition, speech and language, and motor behaviors, a taxonomy of Neurologic Music Therapy techniques has been developed using the standards of best practice.

RATIONALE FOR THE USE OF MUSIC IN THERAPY FOR NEUROLOGIC DISORDERS

Sensorimotor

Epstein (1985) stated that tempo exerts one of the most powerful controls in music, affecting everything that will occur in the performance of a work. He also identified that there is a universal central timing system which enables humans to change tempo proportionally in low integer ratios.

Research by Lang, Obrig, Lindinger, Cheyne, and Deecke (1990) also proposed that there must be a central timing system that drives both the left and right limbs. Both of these studies demonstrate that timing and rhythm have an impact on movement.

Three concepts in motor control provide a good starting point while considering the role of music, particularly rhythm, in movement: sensorimotor control, motor programming, and goal directed movement.

Sensorimotor control refers to how we use sensory input to guide movement. Two principles of rhythmic auditory input related to sensory motor control are priming and timing of the motor response. Considering priming, it is known that at certain intensity levels, acoustic signals can shorten the reaction time of reflex and voluntary movement (Paltsev & Elner, 1967) and can increase physiological muscle activity during H-reflex stimulation (Rossignol & Melvill Jones, 1976). In regard to timing, Rossignol and Melvill Jones found that during a hopping movement performed with an auditory rhythm, the physiological motor events became synchronized to the external pacing signal.

Motor programming is a second concept to consider in relationship to movement and auditory stimulus. Skillful and complex movement is thought to be assembled into programs in the brain as restructured plans which include movement objectives, means of controlling sensorimotor information during the movement, and sets of muscle commands to execute the movement. Rhythm facilitates the development of effective motor programs by organizing movement in anticipatory time, space, and force patterns, therefore making movement trajectories more fluent, smooth, and better timed (Prassas, Thaut, McIntosh, & Rice, 1997).

The third concept to consider in relationship to movement and auditory stimuli, is *goal directed movement.* Organized motor patterns are programmed by goals, not targeted by precise individual movement segments. Since anticipation patterns and temporal targets are intrinsically built into the time structure of music, and these are essential for developing efficient motor patterns, an auditory rhythmic stimulus can act as a timekeeper to reorganize movement by setting a goal in time, space, and force.

An additional concept about the putative role of auditory rhythm in movement facilitation comes from recent studies into rhythmic entrainment and motor synchronization mechanisms. Evidence has emerged that rhythmic motor synchronization is primarily driven by interval adaptation or frequency entrainment rather than event synchronization or phase entrainment between motor response and the rhythmic beat (Thaut, Miller, & Schauer, 1997). When using rhythm in movement cuing, this may mean that time stability is enhanced by rhythmic synchronization throughout the whole duration and trajectory of the movement and not just at the endpoints of the movement coincidental with the rhythmic beat.

The amount of clinical research supporting the use of music in the rehabilitation of movement of both the upper and lower extremities is overwhelming, and very exciting for the field of Neurologic Music Therapy. Several studies have investigated clinically whether auditory rhythm can facilitate gait performance in children with neurological disorders such as cerebral palsy, traumatic brain injuries, and cerebral vascular accidents, all showing significant results supporting the use of rhythm. One notable study published by Thaut, Miller, and Schauer (1998) looked at the effect of rhythmic auditory stimulation on gait patterns of children with spastic diplegic cerebral palsy. Subjects trained with a rhythmic stimulus for 30 minutes a day over a 3-week period. During entrainment of normal walking speed, with a rhythmic stimulus, gait velocity improved in both normal and fast walking speeds. Increases in velocity were attributed to faster cadences and increased stride length. With rhythmic cuing, swing symmetry also improved significantly during both normal and fast-paced walking. It was also noted that daily training with rhythm resulted in increased velocity. Video motion analysis showed kinematic changes of improved knee and hip range of motion as well as smoother knee and hip trajectories. Researchers concluded that children with spastic diplegia were able to entrain to the rhythmic stimulus and demonstrated functional improvements in gait patterns.

Malherbe, Breniere, and Bril (1992) examined how hemiplegic children with cerebral palsy control their gait, emphasizing the capacity of motor-handicapped children to adapt their gait control. He identified rhythmicity and double-support control as the main factors responsible for stability, and consequently recommends that physiotherapy should strive to develop these capacities.

A study by Hurt, Rice, McIntosh, and Thaut (1997) looked at using a rhythmic auditory stimulus in a frequency entrainment design and as a therapeutic stimulus to facilitate gait patterns of 8 traumatically brain injured individuals with persisting gait disorder, 4–24 months post injury. During entrainment, with a rhythmic stimulus with a frequency matched to the subjects baseline cadences, velocity and stride symmetry both increased by an average of 18%. Increases contributing to the velocity improvement were seen in both stride length and cadence as well. When the rhythmic stimulus was accelerated 5% over the fast walking step rate of the subjects, 5 of the subjects were able to entrain to a higher step frequency. The 2 subjects with the slowest baseline gait velocity could not entrain to faster frequencies. After 5 weeks of daily training with a rhythmic stimulus, 5 of the subjects' mean velocity, cadence and symmetry all increased significantly. Improvements in stride symmetry were not statistically significant.

This study offered the first evidence in support of the benefit of using a rhythmic stimulus in the gait training treatment of patients with traumatic brain injuries. The results of the first experiment demonstrated that TBI patients can synchronize their walking patterns to a rhythmic stimulus, although exact entrainment ability seems somewhat deficient and highly variable across different patients probably due to the diffuse and wide spread focus of brain injuries TBI patients endure. The second experiment offered evidence that over time, training with a rhythmic stimulus can result in statistically significant increases in velocity, cadence, and stride length, even when the subject is no longer making progress in conventional physical therapy. The results are specifically interesting because these training effects were achieved with subjects who were all past the initial phase of 3 months, where most spontaneous neurological recovery occurs and therefore the most significant therapy benefits are expected to occur. Thus, these results provide encouraging preliminary evidence that rhythmic cuing can facilitate long-term gait training in TBI patients.

In addition to research examining the effects of auditory rhythm on the lower extremities, Thaut , Schleiffers, and Davis (1991) did a study to analyze auditory rhythm as a time keeper to modify the onset, duration, and variability of electromyographic (EMG) patterns in the biceps and triceps during the performance of a gross motor task. The results indicated a decreased variability in muscle activity during a motor task when auditory rhythm was present, indicating a more efficient recruitment of motor units as necessary in skilled movement. These results may also indicate that more efficient use of the muscles would lead to a patient's ability to endure a task for a longer period of time.

An additional study by Thaut (1985) looked at the use of auditory rhythm and rhythmic speech to aid temporal muscular control in 6–8 year old children with gross motor dysfunction. The results indicated that rhythmic auditory cues and rhythmic speech, used in a motor rhythmic training program, successfully aided temporal muscle control in a complex gross motor sequence. With the use of auditory rhythm and rhythmic speech, the treatment group performed the gross motor task with significantly better motor rhythmic accuracy than did control subjects with only visual modeling.

Speech and Communication Skills

A variety of verbal and nonverbal communication deficits can be seen in children with neurologic disorders, ranging in scope from understanding of spoken language, producing speech, reading and writing, to using a symbol system for communication such as gestures, sign language, or selecting pictures from visual communication charts.

Autistic children can display significant disturbances in their communication skills, often exhibiting a complete absence of desire or ability to communicate verbally or nonverbally with their surroundings. Research shows that only about half of all autistic children will develop functional language ability (Rutter & Bartak, 1973). A few research studies have looked at the use of music to develop acquisition of functional language and communication skills utilizing such mediums as improvisation (Edgerton, 1994; Thaut, 1988).

Apraxia of speech is another common disorder in children which affects motor planning and positioning necessary for voluntary speech. Helfrich-Miller (1984) examined the use of modified Melodic Intonation Therapy (MIT) with developmentally apraxic children. The modified MIT used in the study had three levels instead of the four prescribed by Sparks and Holland (1976). Instead of tapping the rhythm of the phrases as in traditional MIT, the study used sign language to help the subjects recall the words and syntactical structure. The results indicated that MIT can be an effective treatment with developmentally apraxic children.

Although expressive aphasia in children is not very common, some children who have suffered a cerebral vascular accident may present with this impairment of ability to use language. A study by Naeser and Helm-Estabrooks (1985) looked at the CT scans of aphasic cases to see if there was a correspondence between how well a patient responded to MIT and the location of lesions caused by the stroke. The results suggested that patients who respond well to MIT have lesions in Broca's area of the brain, no lesions in Wernicke's area , and no lesions in the right hemisphere. Patients who responded poorly to MIT revealed bilateral lesions, including small right parietal or right frontal lobe lesions, and large lesions in Wernicke's area.

Cognition

Research has revealed several interesting facts related to the organizational processes involved in cognitive musical tasks such as listening, attention, and memory. Although research does suggest some hemispheric dominance for specific musical tasks, such as singing in the right hemisphere, both hemispheres play a significant role in the perception of music. The right brain perceives holistic, spatial, and synthetic relationships, while the left brain is more important in musical punctuation and organization. However, rhythm is one musical element that is processed primarily in both hemispheres (Frisina & Walton, 1988; Zatorre, 1998). A study by Sergent, Zuck, Terriah, and MacDonald (1992) demonstrated that music perception and performance require the activation of many brain areas in both hemispheres as well as lower and higher brain areas, such as the cerebellum, the auditory cortex, the motor cortex, the superior temporal gyrus, the visual cortex, and (unlike language processing) the parietal lobe. These findings show that even though similar brain areas are activated in processing language and music, there are certain distinctions. Music requires different brain circuitry and activates areas not required in language processing. Therefore, with music, the brain functions in a way unlike any other task.

Sloboda (1985) suggested that when listeners perceive music, they start the organizational process by identifying relationships and significant groupings such as gestalt principles, abstractions, and hierarchical structures. In addition, Deutsch (1982) identified the importance of stimulus attributes of music such as frequency, amplitude, and spatial locations, or more complex elements such as timbre.

Numerous studies have been done looking at the effects of music on cognitive learning. Wallace (1994), Gfeller (1983), and Claussen and Thaut (1997) explored musical mnemonics as an organizational process, using grouping or chunking through melodic and rhythmic patterns to assist in text recall with children. The results of their studies indicated that familiar, simple, and repetitive music and rhythmic sequences are all significant elements that contribute to the effectiveness of musical mnemonics as an aide to learning.

Berel, Diller, and Orgel (1971) explored music as an auditory stimulus to aid in a visual motor sequence task in children with cerebral palsy. The results indicated that children more accurately replicated tone sequences when given the auditory stimulus over visual stimulus alone.

Thaut (1988) examined improvised tone sequences of autistic children, as compared to musical improvisations by normal and mentally challenged control subjects. The data indicated that autistic children's tone patterns (analyzed and scored for rhythm, restriction, complexity, rule adherence, and originality) almost reached the scores of normal children and were significantly higher than the control group of mentally challenged individuals. The autistic children's tone sequences showed high scores on the rhythm, restriction, and originality scales, which support the notion of unusual musical responsiveness and abilities in autistic children when compared to results in other performance and behavioral areas.

In a recent study by Thaut and Mahraum (2003), 10 children with a primary diagnosis of autistic disorder and Asperger syndrome performed a task matching visual object cards under three background conditions: (a) silence, (b) auditory rhythmic patterns, and (c) music. In this study, accuracy in a cognitive task, which involved visual object recognition, object matching, and aspects of sustained visual attention, was significantly enhanced in both the auditory rhythm pattern and music conditions. The study also revealed that faster performance times were associated with higher accuracy scores and decreased off-task behaviors in the rhythm and music conditions, but not in the silence condition, suggesting a possible role of rhythm in timing processes of cognitive functions.

Autistic children often present with a wide variety of cognitive deficits. Several studies have looked at the relationship between music and the performance of autistic children on cognitive tasks such as attention (Kostka, 1993), auditory processing (Heaton, Hermelin, & Pring, 1988;

Heaton, Pring, & Hermelin, 2001), affective perception (Heaton, Hermelin, & Pring, 1999), improvisation (Hermelin, O'Connor, Lee, & Treffert, 1989), local and global processing of music (Mottron, Peretz, & Menard, 2000), auditory discrimination (McGivern, Berka, Languis, & Chapman, 1991), and learning and retention of information (Wolfe & Hom, 1993).

GOALS IN NEUROLOGIC MUSIC THERPY WITH CHILDREN

Neurologic music therapy addresses three goal areas in order to increase cognitive, motor, social, communicative, musical and emotional functioning in disabled children: (a) educational, (b) rehabilitative, and (c) developmental (Thaut, 1999). A Neurologic Music Therapist works closely with the interdisciplinary treatment team and must be familiar with developmental, psychological, and medical information that pertains to each disability in order to appropriately address these goals.

Educational goals focus on the academic development of a child. These goals may address social, cognitive, or physical skills. Examples of this may be using a musical mnemonic to teach a child his phone number and address, practicing learning colors and shapes by filling in the blanks of a song, doing creative movement to music, or practicing social skills while participating in a group instrumental playing experience.

Rehabilitative goals work toward restoration or compensatory strategies to improve movement, respiration, posture and sensory perception. For example, using rhythmic auditory stimulation to address gait in a 10-year-old who has developmentally already learned to walk, but recently suffered a traumatic brain injury which has left him with ataxic gait.

Developmental goals strive toward enhancing the normal development of a child by providing normal social, emotional, and sensorimotor experiences through music. Musical experiences are used to submerge the child in normal recreational and leisure experiences that meet the child on their existing functional level, such as teaching a child how to play a musical instrument using adaptive equipment, in order for the child to play in the school orchestra.

TAXONOMY OF NMT TECHNIQUES AS DEFINED IN THE TRAINING MANUAL FOR NEUROLOGIC MUSIC THERAPY (Thaut, 1999)

NMT Sensorimotor Techniques

Neurologic music therapy offers a variety of musical interventions and experiences to address motor skills in physically disabled children. Common goals that are addressed include gait and mobility, strength and endurance, coordination, balance and posture, and range of motion. These goals are addressed through three techniques: Rhythmic Auditory Stimulation (RAS), Patterned Sensory Enhancement (PSE), and Therapeutic Instrumental Music Performance (TIMP).

Rhythmic Auditory Stimulation (RAS) is a neurologic technique used to facilitate the rehabilitation of movements that are intrinsically biologically rhythmical, most importantly gait. RAS uses the physiological effects of auditory rhythm on the motor system to improve the control of movement in rehabilitation of functional, stable and adaptive gait patterns in patients with significant gait deficits due to neurological impairment. RAS can be used in two different ways: (a) as an immediate entrainment stimulus providing rhythmic cues during movement, and (b) as a facilitating stimulus for training in order to achieve more functional gait patterns.

Several variables are important to consider when using RAS with children. Foremost, is to be aware of the sensorimotor developmental stage that the child is in. Research has shown that children under the age of 5 do not reliably entrain to a rhythmic beat (Sloboda, 1985), so depending on the age of the child, a synchronized entrainment to a rhythmic stimulus may not be realistically achievable. This does not preclude the use of RAS with children however. Clinical research has shown that auditory rhythm effects not only temporal organization of gait movements but also spatial control, and thus is thought to act more centrally to mediate changes in motor control (Thaut, Miller & Schauer, 1998).

In addition, Pouthas (1996), in her replicated study to investigate the development of temporal regulations in young children (4–7-year-olds), found that by the end of a fourth training session, children learned to space out their motor responses with a time frame. The researchers concluded that, although this is a skill thought to be acquired at a later stage of ontogenesis, it can be a learned response at an earlier state. This information further confirms the utilization of RAS with young children, however indicates that repeated practice is essential.

When using RAS in the treatment of adult gait disorders, protocol suggests using a process called step-wise limit cycle entrainment (SLICE). Using this optimization strategy, the therapist begins by setting the RAS frequency at the patient's current limit cycle or preferred step cadence. Once the patient has entrained to the rhythmic stimulus, the RAS frequency is increased, working towards approximating the patient's pre-injury step cadence. A more normal gait pattern may result as long as the neurological and mechanical constraints of the motor system are not violated, i.e., the tempo of the RAS must not exceed the patient's capabilities (Thaut et al., 1999.)

However, another factor to be considered when using RAS with young children is that they generally have quite a fast internal cadence. It is important to be familiar with the normal ranges for a child's developmental age before beginning RAS treatment. Though impaired by hemiparesis, children tend to quickly form maladaptive gait patterns to adjust their locomotion speed, probably so they can keep up with their peers. Thus, step-wise limit cycle entrainment is not always appropriate to enhance gait parameters and kinematics in pediatric clients. In many cases rather, it is more appropriate to slow down the cadence of the child and work on specific gait deviations to improve overall ambulation. Most children are not interested in "how" they walk and therefore it can prove challenging to keep a child focused on specific gait training in the clinic. However, the intrinsic properties of the music make it a motivating stimulus to attend to therefore helping a child focus on their gait training.

> *"H" is a 7-year-old girl who experienced an ischemic middle cerebral artery stroke and was following an RAS gait training program to address asymmetry of gait, uneven stance time, ankle circumduction, insufficient dorsiflexion, and inadequate heel strike and arm swing. She had an average cadence that was not terribly different to a "normal" cadence for a child her age; therefore, improving cadence and velocity were not her primary goals, but rather a focus on stride symmetry, heel strike, and arm swing. In addition to the RAS gait training, music therapy sessions focused on pre-gait exercises to increase strength in lower extremities. Later, higher level balance activities were also a part of her therapeutic plans. Upper extremity therapeutic interventions involving gross and fine motor tasks, also were utilized for improved strength, range of motion,*

and to encourage functional use of her affected upper extremities. "H" was asked to practice during the week with her RAS cassette tapes for a home walking program, as well as working with the music therapist and physical therapist utilizing live music facilitation once a week. The results showed measurable improvements in her walking patterns by the end of treatment, even when RAS was not present.

"M" was a 2½-year-old child with cerebral palsy who engaged in an RAS treatment program to address crawling. As with walking, crawling is an intrinsically rhythmic motor movement. It was reasoned, that although the child was developmentally too young to be able to specifically entrain her crawling movements to a rhythmic stimuli, the temporal structure of the music would facilitate a more coordinated physical effort while crawling on the part of the child. No formal kinematic analysis was conducted; however, in video observations, improvements in her timing and her ability to coordinate her ambulation efforts are readily observable.

Patterned Sensory Enhancement (PSE) is a technique which uses the rhythmic, melodic, harmonic and dynamic-acoustical elements of music to provide temporal, spatial, and force cues for movements which reflect functional exercises and activities of daily living. PSE is broader in application than RAS, because it is (a) applied to movements that are not rhythmical by nature (e.g., most arm and hand movements, functional movement sequences such as dressing or sit-to-stand transfers), and (b) it provides more than just temporal cues. PSE uses musical patterns to assemble single, discrete motions (e.g., arm and hand movements during reaching and grasping), into functional movement patterns and sequences. PSE also cues them temporally, spatially, and dynamically during training exercises (Thaut et al., 1991). PSE is often used to work toward goals to increase physical strength and endurance, improve balance and posture, and increase functional motor skills of the upper limbs.

When implementing this technique, it is important to forego the idea of *accompaniment*, and think instead of *sonification*. Too often music therapists accompany themselves and their clients on the guitar or keyboard, providing pleasing background for a song or movement sequence. However, they miss the opportunity to capitalize on manipulating the varied elements of the music in order to musically create the movement by using the spatial, temporal and force cues which are inherent in music. When musical cues are properly used to facilitate rather than accompany movement, clients are better able to organize and respond to motor expectations.

In our clinical work, we have found that the keyboard and the autoharp are the most effective instruments to execute PSE. The range and dynamic capabilities of the keyboard are particularly effective for facilitating complex PSE sequences. The autoharp is also a dynamic and facile therapeutic tool that is often overlooked by music therapist. No other portable instrument is quite able to replicate the spatial and force cueing elements necessary to facilitate motor performance like the autoharp, thus assisting clients in more effective execution of functional exercises and movement patterns.

Therapeutic Instrumental Music Performance (TIMP) is the playing of musical instruments in order to exercise and stimulate functional movement patterns. Appropriate musical instruments are selected in a therapeutically meaningful way in order to emphasize range of motion, endurance, strength, functional hand movements, finger dexterity, and limb coordination (Clark & Chadwick, 1980; Elliott, 1982). During TIMP, instruments are not typically played in the traditional manner, but are placed in different locations to facilitate practice of the desired functional movements. Naturally, instruments are played utilizing adaptive equipment in order to meet the patients' needs and skill level.

In the case of the aforementioned 2½-year-old child with cerebral palsy, there were multiple needs to address for improving her crawling abilities. Crawling requires using a variety of muscles in a coordinated fashion. Weight bearing and weight shifting through the upper and lower extremities is a prerequisite for crawling (Bly, 1994). Abdominal/trunk muscles also play an important role in crawling. Therefore, the main goal areas for treatment were: (a) strengthening her trunk, and, (b) improving strength and timing in her upper extremities. Therapeutic Instrumental Music Performance (TIMP) provided an ideal therapeutic intervention to facilitate the necessary strengthening exercises in which "M" needed to actively participate in order to improve in her ability to crawl. Some examples of the TIMP interventions used with her are as follows: "M" would lay prone in a sling swing and reach up to tap a tambourine as the swing swung forward, thus working on upper back and neck strength; "M" would sit on a therapy ball and reach forward or to the side to play various instruments to increase trunk control and trunk stability. She would lay prone over a foam wedge and reach to play an instrument with one hand while supporting herself with her other hand to increase weight bearing on her upper extremities.

In the case of the previously mentioned 7-year-old girl, a wide variety of TIMP interventions were also utilized to facilitate specific physical goals. Examples include interventions such as kicking the tambourines with her heels while standing (to increase hamstring strength), laying prone on a swing and self-propelling the swing forward with lower extremities to a drum and reaching out with the paretic arm to tap the drum (to increase functional upper extremity use and increase lower extremity strength), utilizing adaptive mallets to strengthen grip and to work on bilateral use of upper extremities while playing drums placed in a circular fashion, working on ankle dorsiflexion by tapping woodblocks suspended above and below "H's" foot with disco taps attached to the bottom and top of her foot.

The possibilities are limitless for creatively challenging children to reach, balance, stretch, and utilize their upper and lower extremities in functional movements with a variety of percussion instruments. The instruments provide a specific target for the children to aim towards. The instruments also define the parameters of the desired movement. For example, if you want a child to work on increasing biceps/triceps strength and elbow range of motion, a woodblock can be placed in the child's lap and another can be held up by the child's shoulder. By tapping one woodblock and then the other, in a repetitive fashion, the child completes the desired exercise movement. Not only do the instruments define the parameters of the movement visually, but the child also receives auditory feedback from successfully hitting the "target" as well as kinesthetic feedback from contacting the mallet with the instrument. Asking a child to play the instruments with you for the duration of a song can be much more motivating than asking them to do 12 biceps curls.

The benefits of utilizing TIMP in therapy sessions is greatly increased by the way in which the neurologic music therapist enhances the client's musical participation with his/her facilitating music. Particularly in the pediatric setting, another key element to successfully implementing NMT techniques is the therapist's ability to simplify and readily adapt to the functional level of the child. Simple, repetitive melodies, familiar or not, have been most successful with our clients. It is a common failing in much of the prerecorded and/or written pediatric music, to try to utilize clever and too complicated lyrics. The music therapist's ability to distill the lyrics to an appropriate vocabulary level, or simply create their own, more appropriate musical compositions, leads to much more effective interaction with children of all functional levels.

NMT Speech Techniques

Neurologic Music Therapy can play a large role in the development and rehabilitation of both verbal and nonverbal communication skills in children. NMT has eight techniques which address speech disorders, based on the current research in this area. Techniques in NMT can be used to address disorders such as: apraxia; fluency disorders such as stuttering and cluttering; aphasia; and voice disorders which may result in abnormal pitch, loudness, timbre, breath control, or prosody of speech. Goals in the area of speech and communication address issues such as functional and spontaneous speech, speech comprehension, motor control and coordination essential for articulation, fluency of speech, vocal production and sequencing of speech sounds, and rate and intelligibility. When working with children it is especially important to be aware of their developmental stage when choosing a technique that would best address their current needs.

Melodic Intonation Therapy (MIT) is a treatment technique developed for expressive aphasia rehabilitation which utilizes a patient's unimpaired ability to sing, to facilitate spontaneous and voluntary speech through sung and chanted melodies which resemble natural speech intonation patterns (Sparks, Helm, & Albert, 1974). When using MIT with aphasia, the emphasis is to increase the linguistic or semantic aspects of verbal utterances. Although it is very unusual for children to present with expressive aphasia, therapists have also used this techniques as a more phonetical intervention for verbal apraxia.

It is important to remember that this MIT is only appropriate for a very small patient population; however, it can be very effective when appropriately applied. Since the MIT protocol is very specific and requires a patient to be seen over an extended period of time (6 or more months), modified versions of this technique have also proven to be effective with acute patients as long as the seven principles of language therapy involved in MIT are maintained.

Speech Stimulation (STIM) is the use of musical materials such as songs, rhymes, chants, and musical phrases simulating prosodic speech gestures to stimulate nonpropositional speech. STIM uses completion or initiation of overlearned familiar song lyrics, association of words with familiar tunes, or musical phrases to elicit functional speech responses (Basso, Capitani, & Vigndo, 1979). For example, spontaneous completion of familiar sentences is stimulated through familiar tunes or obvious melodic phrases (e.g., "You are my _____", or "How are you _____?"). MSS is most often used with apraxic and aphasic patients. It can be used as a follow up to Melodic Intonation Therapy in order to increase the number of functional verbal utterances that a patient is able to produce (e.g., " I want _____" or "I don't want _____").

> *"D" is an 8-year-old autistic boy who has limited propositional speech and frequently demonstrates echolalic speech patterns. Speech Stimulation is being used during music therapy sessions to increase "D's" propositional speech. During initial assessment he was able to identify a great number of picture icons, but was unable to use this information in any meaningful way. Through utilization of the technique of Speech Stimulation, "D" has progressed from simple naming of pictures, to singing the phrase "I see a _____," and finally on to singing a more complex phrase: "I see a ________, and the __________ _________." (e.g. "I see a frog, and the frog jumps.") The final stage of "D's" progress with this technique has been to fade out the music and have him say the sentences. We are continuing to make progress in transferring this sentence structure into spontaneous speech for "D."*
>
> *"D" also has mastered the phrase "I want to play the _______." Throughout treatment sessions he is now able to verbalize his request for an instrument rather than grabbing what he wants.*

Rhythmic Speech Cuing (RSC) is the use of rhythmic cuing to control the initiation and rate of speech thru cuing and pacing. The therapist may use the client's hand, a drum, or possibly a metronome to prime speech patterns or pace the rate of speech. This technique can be useful to facilitate motor planning for an apraxic patient, cue muscular coordination for dysarthria, or assist in pacing with fluency disorders.

> *A 10- year-old, autistic client, "B," speaks very rapidly, and is frequently unintelligible because of this accelerated rate. By practicing key phrases utilizing Rhythmic Speech Cuing with a drum, "B" is able to imitate a more appropriate rate of speech and therefore be understood. The therapist initially taps the appropriate rhythm of the sentence on the drum, then "B" echoes this pattern. The therapist then taps and says the sentence simultaneously—then "B" repeats this. The sentence is repeated numerous times in this way until "B" achieves intelligibility. "B" then says the sentence without the drumming. As "B" becomes proficient with a sentence, the drum is utilized less and less. "B" has actually begun to self-cue his speech by simply tapping his finger on his leg as a reminder of the slower pacing.*

Vocal Intonation Therapy (VIT) is the use of intoned phrases simulating the prosody, inflection, and pacing of normal speech. This is done through vocal exercises which train all aspects of voice control including: inflection, pitch, breath control, timbre, and dynamics. An example would be to sing a five-note scale and gradually move the starting pitch up or down by half steps with a child who has a limited pitch range in their normal speaking voice. This exercise could be further expanded by adding a functional sentence, i.e., "Let's go out and play."

Therapeutic Singing (TS) is a technique which involves the unspecified use of singing activities to facilitate initiation, development, and articulation in speech and language as well as to increase functions of the respiratory apparatus. Therapeutic singing can be used with a variety of neurological or developmental speech and language dysfunctions (Glover, Kalinowski, Rastatter, & Stuart, 1996; Jackson, Treharne, & Boucher, 1997).

Oral Motor and Respiratory Exercises (OMREX) involves the use of musical materials and exercises, mainly through sound vocalization and wind instrument playing, to enhance articulatory control and respiratory strength and function of the speech apparatus. This technique would be used with such populations as developmental disorders, dysarthria, and muscular dystrophy (Haas, Distenfeld, & Axen, 1986).

> *In cooperative sessions with speech therapy, 9-year-old "K" began treatment after receiving a cochlear implant. In addition to her hearing impairment, "K" also had an extreme overbite and protruding front teeth that prevented her from attaining proper lip closure for articulation. Two versions of OMREX were used to address this problem. "K" would imitate various sounds (targeted by the speech therapist) within the context of a specific call and response song the therapist composed for her. In this way "P" would specifically practice lip closure, etc., numerous times within the context of her song. "P" also learned to play the kazoo within the context of a specific song which required her to maintain lip closure on the kazoo for longer and longer periods of time.*

Developmental Speech and Language Training Through Music (DSLM) is the specific use of developmentally appropriate musical materials and experiences to enhance speech and language development through singing, chanting, playing musical instruments, and combining music, speech and movement.

> *A multidisciplinary pediatrics group for developmentally delayed 2–5-year-old children addresses motor skills, speech and language development and various other developmental goals through the combination of movement to music, instrumental activities, and singing. The group begins with the children taking turns strumming the autoharp in order to address the development of fine and gross motor skills of the upper extremities. In addition, the children are singing a song which incorporates the names of each group member to work on increasing vocal output and promoting social/pragmatic skills as they take turns passing the pick to one another and saying each other's names. This is only one example of how DSLM is incorporated on a regular basis within this group. All gross motor activities are facilitated with live music to enhance the motor responses of the children, often within the context of a song that gives simple directions or imparts thematic information. Concepts for language development are incorporated within instrumental activities such as matching instruments to instruments or pictures to instruments while identifying similarities and differences. The possibilities for DSLM in this type of group are all but limitless!*

Symbolic Communication Training Through Music (SYCOM) is the use of musical performance exercises using structured instrumental or vocal improvisation to train communication behavior, language pragmatics, appropriate speech gestures, emotional communication in nonverbal language system, that is sensory structured, has strong affective saliency, and can simulate communication structures in social interaction patterns in real time.

NMT Cognitive Techniques

Several Neurologic Music Therapy techniques have been developed to address cognitive learning in children, based on the previously mentioned studies which provide evidence for clinical support in the role of music to aid in memory, attention, and executive function training. Three areas are addressed in cognitive training techniques: Auditory Attention and Perception Training, Memory Training, and Executive Function Training.

Auditory Attention and Perception Training Techniques

Musical Sensory Orientation Training (MSOT) is the use of music, presented live or recorded, to stimulate arousal and recovery of wake states and facilitate meaningful responsiveness and orientation to time, place, and person. In more advanced recovery of developmental stages, training would involve active engagement in simple musical exercises to increase vigilance and train basic attention maintenance with emphasis on quantity rather than quality of response (Ogata, 1995).

> *First seen in the Intensive Care Unit following a major Traumatic Brain Injury, 4-year-old "C" was unresponsive to external stimuli, except for pain. "C's" initial response to music was to noticeably calm. "C's" heart rate and blood pressure readings would immediately lower when live, gentle music and singing was presented to him.*
>
> *After several weeks of developing an increasingly stable physical state, "C" moved to the pediatrics unit where he was seen in co-operative therapy sessions with Occupational Therapy. "C" would resist OT's attempts to provide range of motion to his upper extremities, but when the OT would assist "C" in strumming the autoharp and the music therapist would sing "Cs" favorite song, the tone in his upper extremities would noticeably decrease and the OT would be able to prompt "C" in various instrumental music interventions. As these sessions continued, "C" began to briefly open his eyes and also show more muscular responses with less prompting from the OT.*

Musical Neglect Training (MNT) involves active performance exercises on musical instruments, which are structured in time, tempo, and rhythm, with an appropriate spatial configuration of instruments to focus attention to neglected or unattended visual field. Musical Neglect Training may also involve receptive music listening to stimulate hemispheric brain arousal while engaging in exercises addressing visual neglect or inattention (Anderson & Phelps, 2001; Hommel, et al., 1990).

Auditory Perception Training (APT) is the use of musical exercises to discriminate and identify different components of sound, such as time, tempo, duration, pitch, timbre, rhythmic patterns, as well as speech sounds. Integration of different sensory modalities such as visual, tactile, and kinesthetic input are used during active musical exercises such as playing from symbolic or graphic notion, using tactile sound transmission, or integrating movement to music (Bettison, 1996: Gfeller, Woodworth, Robin, Witt, & Knutson, 1997; Heaton et al., 1988).

Musical Attention Control Training (MACT) involves structured active or receptive musical exercises, using precomposed performance or improvisation, in which musical elements cue different musical responses in order to practice sustained, selective, divided, and alternating attention functions (Thaut, 2003).

> *"J," a 16-year-old boy severally injured in a car accident, was particularly responsive to the various attention control exercises presented to him in individual treatment session during his recovery. Initially "J" was unable to focus his attention on the music therapist's cues. However, he was motivated by his desire to play the pitched*

percussion instruments and various drums and showed daily improvement in his ability to sustain his attention and play instruments according to therapist instructions. By the end of 1 week, "J" was able to sustain his attention within a musical task greater than 5 minutes, as well as demonstrate the ability to attend to alternating music stimuli and respond accordingly to predetermined instructions.

Memory Training Techniques

Musical Mnemonics Training (MMT) is the use of musical exercises to address various memory encoding and decoding/recall functions. Immediate recall of sounds or sung words using musical stimuli may be used to address echoic functions. Musical stimuli may be used as a mnemonic device or memory template in a song, rhyme, chant, or to facilitate learning of nonmusical information by sequencing and organizing the information in temporally structured patterns or chunks (Deutsch, 1982; Gfeller, 1983; Wallace, 1994; Claussen & Thaut, 1997; Maeller, 1996).

Associative Mood and Memory Training (AMMT) involves musical mood induction techniques to instate (a) a mood congruent mood state to facilitate memory recall, or (b) to access associative mood and memory function through inducing a positive emotional state in the learning and recall process (Bower, 1981; Dolan, 2002).

Executive Functioning Training Techniques

Musical Executive Function Training (MEFT) is the use of improvisation and composition exercises in a group or individually to practice executive function skills such as organization, problem solving, decision-making, reasoning, and comprehension, within a social context that provides important therapeutic elements such as performance products in real time, temporal structure, creative process, affective content, sensory structure, and social interaction patterns (Dolan, 2002).

Socioemotional

Disabled children have the same need for healthy emotional and social development and opportunities to express their feelings as do normal children. Because of the experiences of their disabilities, these children may actually have an increased need to cope with feelings, such as grief, depression, or loneliness (Thaut, 1999). On the other hand, they may also be withdrawn socially, causing them to miss out on the support systems that develop through peer relationships. A combination of a lack of ability to participate in some of the more traditional channels to express emotions and a decreased social support system can become a real dilemma for these children.

Although NMT techniques do not specifically addressed socioemotional issues, music can provide an effective medium to create rewarding social and emotional experiences for children. In addition to working on physical, sensory, cognitive or speech goals, music can also help to increase self-esteem and provide an outlet for emotional expression through success-oriented experiences at any level of functioning. Music can also be used in a group setting to provide opportunities for peer interaction and support. Learning how to enjoy the recreational use of music or even developing a life long musical skill such as playing an instrument are also important in the overall strategy to normalize the life of a disabled child.

CONCLUSION

In conclusion, Neurologic Music Therapy is the therapeutic application of music to cognitive, sensory, and motor dysfunction, based on scientific and clinical research. NMT is based on the Standards of Best Practice and the Rational Scientific Mediating Model (R-SMM), a neuroscience model of music perception and production and the influence of music on functional changes in nonmusical brain and behavior function. Due to the strong scientific foundation, NMT provides the framework to systematically and creatively transform musical behaviors into therapeutic behaviors producing consistent and functional results. With the proper training in NMT and the proper assessment, the extensive taxonomy of techniques in NMT makes it easy for trained neurologic music therapist to select the most appropriate therapeutic application and predict the therapeutic outcomes and benefits for their clients.

REFERENCES

Anderson, A. K. & Phelps, E. A. (2001). Lesions of the human amygdala impair enhanced perception of emotionally salient events. *Nature, 411*, 305–309.

Basso, A., Capitani, E., & Vigndo, L. S. (1979). The influence of rehabilitation on language skills in aphasic patients. *Archives of Neurology, 36,* 190–196.

Berel, M., Diller, L., & Orgel, M. (1971). Music as a facilitator for visual motor sequencing tasks in children with cerebral palsy. *Developmental Medicine and Child Neurology, 13,* 335–342.

Berlyne, D. E. (1971). Emotion and arousal. *Aesthetics and Psychobiology* (pp. 61–74). New York: Appleton-Century-Crofts.

Bettison, S. (1996). The long-term effects of auditory training on children with autism. *Journal of Autism and Developmental Disorders, 26,* 361–375.

Bly, L. (1994). *Motor skills acquisition in the first year: An illustrated guide to normal development.* Tucson, AZ: Therapy Skill Builders.

Bower, G. H. (1981). Mood and memory. *American Psychologist, 36*(2), 129–148.

Center for Biomedical Research in Music (CBRM). (1999). *Training manual for Neurologic Music Therapy.* Fort Collins, CO: Colorado State University.

Clark, C., & Chadwick, D. (1980).*Clinically adapted instruments for the multiply handicapped.* St. Louis, MO: Magnamusic-Baton.

Claussen, D. W., & Thaut, M. H. (1997). Music as a mnemonic device for children with learning disabilities. *Canadian Journal of Music Therapy, 5,* 55–56.

Deutsch, D. (1982). Organizational processes in music. In M. Clynes (Ed.), *Music, mind and brain* (pp. 119–131). New York: Plenum Press.

Dolan, R. J. (2002). Emotion, cognition, and behavior. *Science, 298*, 1191–1194.

Edgerton, C. (1994). The effect of improvisational music therapy on the communicative behavior of autistic children. *Journal of Music Therapy, 31*, 31–62.

Elliott, B., (1982). *Guide to the selection of musical instruments with respect to physical ability and disability.* Saint Louis, MO: MMB Music.

Epstein, D. (1985). Tempo relations: A cross-cultural study. *Music Theory Spectrum, 7,* 34–71.

Frisina, R. D., & Walton, J. P. (1988). Neural basis for music cognition: Neurophysiological foundations. *Psychomusicology, 7*, 99–107.

Gfeller, K. (1983). Musical mnemonics as an aid to retention with normal and learning disabled students. *Journal of Music Therapy, 20*, 179–189.

Gfeller, K., Woodworth, G., Robin, D. A., Witt, S., & Knutson, J. F. (1997). Perception of rhythmic and sequential pitch patterns by normally hearing adults and adult cochlear implant users. *Ear and Hearing, 18*, 252–260.

Glover, H., Kalinowski, J., Rastatter, M., & Stuart, A. (1996). Effect of instruction to sing on stuttering frequency at normal and fast rates. *Perceptual and Motor Skills, 83*, 511–522.

Haas, F., Distenfeld, S., & Axen, K. (1986). Effects of perceived music rhythm on respiratory patterns. *Journal of Applied Physiology, 61*, 1185–1191.

Heaton, P., Hermelin, B., & Pring, L. (1988). Autism and pitch processing: A precursor for savant musical ability? *Music Perception, 15*, 291–305.

Heaton, P., Hermilin, B., & Pring, L. (1999). Can children with autistic spectrum disorders perceive affect in music? An experimental investigation. *Psychological Medicine, 29*(6), 1405–1410.

Heaton, P., Pring, L., & Hermelin, B. (2001). Musical processing in high functioning children with autism. *Annals of the New York Academy of Sciences, 930*, 443–444.

Helfrich-Miller, K. R. (1984). Melodic intonation therapy with developmentally apraxic children. *Seminars in Speech and Language, 5*, 119–126.

Hermelin, B., O'Connor, N., Lee, S., & Treffert, D. (1989). Intelligence and musical improvisation. *Psychological Medicine, 19*(2), 447–457.

Hommel, M., Peres, B., Pollak, P., Memin, B., Besson, G., Gaio, J., & Perret, J. (1990). Effects of passive tactile and auditory stimuli on left visual neglect. *Archives of Neurology, 47*, 573–576.

Hurt, C. P., Rice, R. R., McIntosh, G. C., & Thaut, M. H. (1998). Rhythmic auditory stimulation in gait training for patients with traumatic brain injury. *Journal of Music Therapy, 35*, 228–241.

Jackson, S. A., Treharne, D. A., & Boucher, J. (1997). Rhythm and language in children with moderate learning difficulties. *European Journal of Disorders of Communication, 32*, 99–108.

Kostka, M. (1993). A comparison of selected behaviors of a student with autism in special education and regular music class. *Music Therapy Perspectives, 11*, 57–60.

Lang, W., Obrig, H., Lindinger, G., Cheyne, D., & Deecke, L. (1990). Supplementary motor area activation while tapping bimanually different rhythms in musicians. *Experimental Brain Research, 79*, 504–514.

Maeller, D. H. (1996). *Rehearsal strategies and verbal working memory in multiple sclerosis.* Unpublished master's thesis, Colorado State University, Fort Collins.

Malherbe, V., Breniere, Y., & Bril, B. (1992). How do cerebral palsied children with hemiplegia control their gait? In M. Woollacott & F. Horak (Eds.), *Posture and gait: Control mechanisms* (pp. 102–105). Eugene, OR: University of Oregon Books.

McGivern, R. F., Berka, C., Languis, M. L., & Chapman, S. (1991). Detection of deficits in temporal pattern discrimination using the Seashore Rhythm Test in young children with reading impairments. *Journal of Learning Disabilities, 24*, 58–62.

Mottron, L., Peretz, I., & Menard, E. (2000). Local and global processing of music in high-functioning persons with autism: Beyond central coherence. *Journal of Child Psychology and Psychiatry, 41*(8), 1057–1065.

Naeser, M. A., & Helm-Estabrooks, N. (1985). CT scan lesion localization and response to Melodic Intonation Therapy with nonfluent aphasia cases. *Cortex, 21*, 203–223.

Ogata, D. (1995). Human EEG responses to classical music and simulated white noise: Effects of a musical loudness component on consciousness. *Perceptual and Motor Skills, 80*, 779–790.

Paltsev, Y. I., & Elner, A. M. (1967). Change in the functional state of the segmental apparatus of the spinal cord under the influence of sound stimuli and its role in voluntary movement. *Biophysics , 12*, 1219–1226.

Parsons, L. M., & Thaut, M. H. (2001). Functional neuroanatomy of musical rhythm perception. *Journal of Cognitive Neuroscience* (Suppl.), Cognitive Neuroscience Society 8th Annual Conference, *84*.

Pouthas, V. (1996). The development of the perception of time and temporal regulation of action in infants and children. In I. Deliege & J. Sloboda (Eds.), *Musical beginnings: Origins and development of musical dompetence* (pp. 115–141). New York: Oxford University Press.

Pouthas, V., & Jacquet, A. (1987). A developmental study of timing behavior in 4½ and 7-year-old children. *Journal of Experimental Child Psychology*, 43, 282–299.

Prassas, S. G., Thaut, M. H., McIntosh, G. C., & Rice, R. R. (1997). Effect of auditory rhythmic cuing on gait kinematic parameters in stroke patients. *Gait and Posture, 6*, 218–223.

Rossignol, S., & Melvill Jones, G. (1976). Audio-spinal influences in man studied by the H-reflex and its possible role in rhythmic movements synchronized to sound. *Electroencephalography and Clinical Neurophysiology, 41*, 83–92.

Rutter, M., & Bartak, L. (1973). Special educational treatment of autistic children: a comparative study. II. Follow-up findings and implications for services. *Journal of Child Psychology and Psychiatry, 14*, 241–270.

Sergent, J., Zuck, E., Terriah, S., & MacDonald, B. (1992). Distributed neural network underlying musical sight-reading and keyboard performance. *Science, 257*, 106–109.

Sloboda, J. A. (1985). *The musical mind: The cognitive psychology of music*. Oxford: Clarendon Press.

Sparks, R. W., Helm, N., & Albert, M. (1974). Aphasia rehabilitation resulting from melodic intonation therapy. *Cortex, 10*, 313–316.

Sparks, R. W., & Holland, A. L. (1976). Method: Melodic intonation therapy for aphasia. *Journal of Speech and Hearing Disorders, 41*, 298–300.

Stephan, K. M., Thaut, M. H., Wunderlich, G., Schicks, W., Tellmann, L., Herzog, H., McIntosh, G., Seitz, R., Hoemberg, V., & Tian, B. (1999). Rhythmic auditory tracking: Evidence for three distinct cerebellar circuits. *Proceeding of the Society for Neuroscience*, 148.10.

Thaut, M. H. (1985). The use of auditory rhythm and rhythmic speech to aid temporal muscular control in children with gross motor dysfunction. *Journal of Music Therapy, 22*(3), 108–128.

Thaut, M. H. (1987). Visual versus auditory (musical) stimulus preference in autistic children. *Journal of Autism and Developmental Disorders, 17*, 425–432.

Thaut, M. H. (1988). Measuring musical responsiveness in autistic children: A comparative analysis of improvised musical tone sequences of autistic, normal, and mentally retarded individuals. *Journal of Autism and Developmental Disorders, 18*, 561–571.

Thaut, M. H. (1999). Music therapy for children with physical disabilities. In W. B. Davis, K. E. Gfeller, & M. H. Thaut (Eds.), *An introduction to music therapy, theory and practice* (pp. 148–162). Boston: McGraw-Hill.

Thaut, M. H. (2000). *A scientific model of music in therapy and medicine*. St. Louis, MO: MMB Music.

Thaut, M. H., Hurt, C. P., Dragan, D.,& McIntosh, G. C. (1998). Rhythmic entrainment of gait patterns in children with cerebral palsy. *Developmental Medicine and Child Neurology, 40*(78), 15.

Thaut, M. H., Hurt, C. P., & McIntosh, G. C. (1997). Rhythmic entrainment of gait patterns in traumatic brain injury rehabilitation [Abstract]. *Journal of Neurologic Rehabilitation, 11*, 131.

Thaut, M. H., Kenyon, G. P., Schauer, M. L., & McIntosh, G. C. (1999). Rhythmicity and brain function: Implication for therapy of movement disorders. *IEEE Engineering in Medicine and Biology, 18*, 101–108.

Thaut, M. H., & Mahraum, D. (2003). Rhythm enhances cognitive performance in children with autism and Asperger's syndrome: Preliminary evidence. Submitted for publication.

Thaut, M. H., Miller, R. A., & Schauer, M. L. (1997). Rhythm in human motor control: Adaptive mechanisms in movement synchronization. In D. J. Schneck & J. K. Schneck (Eds.), *Music in human adaptation*. Blacksburg, VA: Virginia Polytechnic Institute and State University, 191–198.

Thaut, M. H., Miller R. A., & Schauer, L. M. (1998). Multiple synchronization strategies in rhythmic sensorimotor tasks: Phase versus period adaptation. *Biological Cybernetics, 79*, 241–250.

Thaut, M. H., Schleiffers, S., & Davis, W. B. (1991). Analysis of EMG activity in biceps and triceps muscle in a gross motor task under the influence of auditory rhythm. *Journal of Music Therapy, 28*, 64–88.

Wallace, W. T. (1994). Memory for music: Effect of melody on recall of text. *Journal of Experimental Psychology: Learning, Memory, Cognition, 20*, 1471–1485.

Wolfe, D. E., & Hom, C. (1993). Use of melodies as structural prompts for learning and retention of sequential verbal information by preschool students. *Journal of Music Therapy, 30*, 100–118.

Zatorre, R. J. (1998). Functional specialization of human auditory cortex for musical processing. *Brain, 121*, 1817–1818.

SIX

Coping and Chronic Illness: Music Therapy for Children and Adolescents With Cancer[1]

Sheri L. Robb, Ph.D., MT-BC

MEDICAL PROFESSIONALS and consumers have witnessed dramatic changes in pediatric health care over the last 50 years. Pediatric health care facilities have moved from full exclusion of families to a family-centered health care approach addressing the physical and psychosocial needs of children and their families (Ack, 1993; Perrin, 1993; Siegel & Hudson, 1992). Early studies documenting children's responses to the hospital environment and identifying specific sources of distress are responsible for these changes and have increased the availability of psychosocial interventions—including music therapy for hospitalized children and their families.

Healthcare professionals and administrators recognize that long-term or repeated hospitalizations can have deleterious effects on child development, quality of life, psychological well-being, and/or family functioning. Professionals also recognize that psychosocial problems related to a cancer diagnosis can contribute to the incidence of treatment noncompliance, increased symptom distress, and long-term psychological adjustment (Frank, Blount, & Brown, 1997; Koocher, 1986; Lauria, Hockenberry-Eaton, Pawletko, & Mauer, 1996; Leitenberg, Greenwald, & Cado, 1992; Roth & Newman, 1991; Rourke, Stuber, Hobbie, & Kazak, 1999). Despite admirable gains in the availability of psychosocial interventions and programming, administrators are still faced with having to justify the cost of these treatments and therapies. This requires that medical disciplines demonstrate the efficacy of specific treatments through research and clinical documentation.

Research literature investigating the impact of cancer on children and families have clearly established the need for interventions that promote the acquisition and use of adaptive coping strategies that serve to reduce the impact of prolonged stress associated with a chronic illness and its impending treatment. Coping is a complex interaction of environmental, familial, developmental, and disease-specific variables. Effective music interventions are developed based on a thorough understanding of these variables and how music can be used to alter stress

---

[1]Portions of this article are reprinted, with permission, from *Music Therapy Perspectives,* American Music Therapy Association, Inc. (Robb, 2003).

appraisals and promote the use of adaptive coping skills in patients and their families.

The prevalence of live, interactive music interventions is evident when surveying the pediatric music therapy research literature (Standley & Whipple, 2003). Robertson (1992) surveyed pediatric music therapists and found that live music-making, including singing familiar songs and instrumental improvisation, were among the techniques therapist used most frequently. Singing, playing instruments, musical improvisation, song writing, action songs, and music video production all characterize interventions involving the creation of music. Active music interventions are documented in 21 professional publications (Bailey, 1984; Barrickman, 1989; Brodsky, 1989; Christenberry, 1979; Daveson, 2001; Edwards, 1998; Fagen, 1982; Froehlich, 1996; Hilliard, 2001; Kennelly, 2001; Lindsay, 1981; Loewy, 1997; Malone, 1996; McDonnell, 1983, 1984; Pratt, 1997; Robb, 1996; Robb & Ebberts, 2003a, 2003b; Rudenberg & Royka, 1989; Slivka & Magill, 1986; Standley & Hanser, 1995; Whipple, 2000). Empirical investigations of active music interventions to help children cope with hospitalization are emerging, with approximately 10 studies.

These initial studies indicate that participatory music sessions have proven beneficial in altering mood states (Bailey, 1983; Osborn, 1997), increasing verbalizations about illness (Froehlich, 1984), increasing IgA levels in saliva (Lane, 1991), decreasing distress behaviors related to needle insertions (Malone, 1996), decreasing distress behaviors of infants and toddlers (Marley, 1984), increasing parent–neonate interactions (Whipple, 2000), and reducing grief symptoms in bereaved children (Hilliard, 2001). Additionally, Standley and Whipple's (2003) meta-analysis indicates that live music interventions provided by a trained music therapist resulted in greater benefit than interventions that used recorded music.

Additional music therapy studies have examined two specific treatment protocols that proved effective in promoting increased levels of behavioral engagement, diminishing state anxiety, and promoting communication about concerns related to illness (Robb, 2000; Robb & Ebberts, 2003a; 2003b). These interventions were designed based on a contextual support model of music therapy (Robb, 2000, 2003) which takes into account aspects of hospitalization and cancer treatment that are stressful for children, the relationship between coping and development, and the proposed mechanisms by which music can be used to create supportive environments and promote active engagement during times of stress. This chapter begins by identifying the critical needs of children and adolescents who have been diagnosed with cancer.

CHILDREN WITH CANCER: THE CRITICAL NEED FOR COPING INTERVENTIONS

Advances in pediatric cancer treatment are responsible for the increased number of children who now survive, experiencing either complete or prolonged disease remission. Despite these advances, cancer continues to be the second leading cause of death among children between the ages of 1 and 14 in the United States. According to statistics compiled by the American Cancer Society in 2003, the incidence of childhood cancer has stabilized since the late 1980s and mortality rates have steadily declined since 1975, with 5-year relative survival rates among children for all cancer types improving from 56% in the mid 1970s to 77% in 1990s (Jemal et al., 2003).

The growing number of childhood cancer survivors has raised concerns regarding delayed effects of the disease on psychological and physiological functioning (Rowland, 1990). Research has made it increasingly clear that many children and adolescents do not have a sufficient repertoire of illness-related coping strategies to buffer the impact of a cancer diagnosis and resulting treatment. A growing body of research indicates that children who are exposed to life-threatening illnesses are at risk for developing symptoms of posttraumatic stress disorder (Rourke et al., 1999; Stuber, Shemesh, & Saxe, 2003), depressive symptoms (Kaplan, Busner, Weinhold, & Lenon, 1987; Kusch, Labouvie, Ladisch, Fleischhack, & Bode, 2000), and diminished life quality (Grootenhuis & Last, 2001). Inadequate or maladaptive coping in pediatric patients has also been associated with treatment noncompliance (Tebbi, 1993), increased symptom distress including anxiety, pain, fatigue, and mood (Lauria et al., 1996; Koocher, 1986), developmental regression (Lauria et al., 1996), and poorer treatment outcomes (Broers et al., 1998; Loberiza et al., 2002; Molassiotis, Van Den Akker, Milligan, & Goldman, 1997; Tschuschke, Hertenstein, Arnold, Bunjes, & Denzinger, 2001).

Given that the emotional problems of children with cancer do not necessarily diminish over time, researchers and clinicians advocate a preventative approach to psychosocial intervention (Grootenhuis & Last, 2001; Zebrack & Chelser, 2002). In support of a preventative approach, Kusch and colleagues (2000) cite evidence that successful coping experiences in the initial treatment phase for cancer are related to better emotional adjustment and coping during subsequent phases of treatment. Further support for a preventative approach can be found in studies that have consistently shown an association between the use of active coping strategies and diminished levels of distress and adjustment problems, whereas the prolonged use of avoidant coping strategies is associated with increased levels of distress and adjustment problems (Leitenberg et al., 1992; Roth & Newman, 1991; Trask et al., 2003). Based on their findings that a strong relationship exists between the increased use of active coping strategies and lower distress in adolescent patients with cancer, Trask and colleagues (2003) call for interventions that aim to increase the use of engagement coping strategies to facilitate adjustment to cancer. As such, this chapter focuses on music therapy interventions used during acute periods of cancer treatment where the purpose of interventions are to identify and promote the use of adaptive coping strategies and increase communication among patients, families, and healthcare providers.

COPING AND SELF-REGULATION

The contextual support model of music therapy is a developing theory that seeks to describe and investigate the mechanisms that are responsible for bringing about changes in self-regulatory behaviors during times of stress. To date, this model has been based primarily on the motivational model of coping proposed by Skinner and Wellborn (1994). This motivational model of coping examines coping as a function of behavior regulation. Theorists argue that humans have fundamental psychological needs for competence, autonomy, and relatedness to others. Skinner and Wellborn (1994) maintain that the drive to fulfill these three psychological needs influence and direct an individual's behavior. The authors also discuss attributes of the environment and the self that contribute to an individual's stress appraisal and resulting action.

Coping researchers are also investigating the critical role that attention and emotions play in the processes of stress appraisal and self-regulation. Wilson and Gottman (1996) argue that attentional processes serve as a shuttle between cognitive and emotional functioning. These authors describe the impact of stress on attentional processes and how an individual's ability to shift and maintain attentional focus is fundamental to the process of emotional regulation. Similarly, attention and coping assume central roles in Compas and Boyer's (2001) biopsychosocial model of children's health. Based on clinical observations and research outcomes, it has become increasingly clear that emotion regulation and attention must be more fully integrated into the contextual support model of music therapy. Although attributes of the environment, traits of the child, and development are critical to understanding and developing effective music interventions, equal attention must be given to the role of emotion and attention. Given that music has been found to have a significant impact on emotions and attentional behaviors, it is probable that a closer examination of these variables will improve our understanding of how music can be used to modify stress appraisals and coping responses.

In the sections that follow, the author first provides an overview of the contextual support model of music therapy as originally proposed—highlighting the importance of environmental and personal attributes that contribute to stress appraisals. Second, that author addresses developmental issues that directly influence coping strategies used by children and adolescents and how music therapy interventions are used to support these developmental changes. The final section of the chapter will provide an overview of research concerning the role of attention and emotion in stress appraisal and self-regulation—calling for revisions to the original model.

A CONTEXTUAL SUPPORT MODEL OF MUSIC THERAPY

Despite improved availability of psychosocial programs for hospitalized children, the environment remains a potential source of stress for children and their families. Invasive procedures, unfamiliar and isolated environments, and separation from family and friends are often unavoidable realities of hospitalization that can contribute to children's stress appraisals. The challenge is to find ways to motivate children to be active participants in an environment that often encourages passivity.

The contextual support model of music therapy is based on Skinner and Wellborn's (1994) proposition that contextual support (e.g., structure, autonomy support, and involvement) influence coping in two ways. First, contextual support buffers the effects of stress, reducing the psychological distress experienced by children. Second, contextual support can influence the way a child copes. Increased structure is hypothesized to result in more active behavior, more autonomy support to increase self-determined behaviors, and increased availability of social support to increase the child's use of that support. The aim of the music therapy intervention, therefore, is to reengage children with their environment using music to create three elements of contextual support: (a) Structure: to provide children with opportunities for successful mastery over the environment, (b) Autonomy Support: to afford children opportunities to make choices and direct activities, and (c) Involvement: to express unconditional acceptance of children and reinforce their efforts and actions.

The contextual support model of music therapy, illustrated in Figure 1, can be summarized as follows:

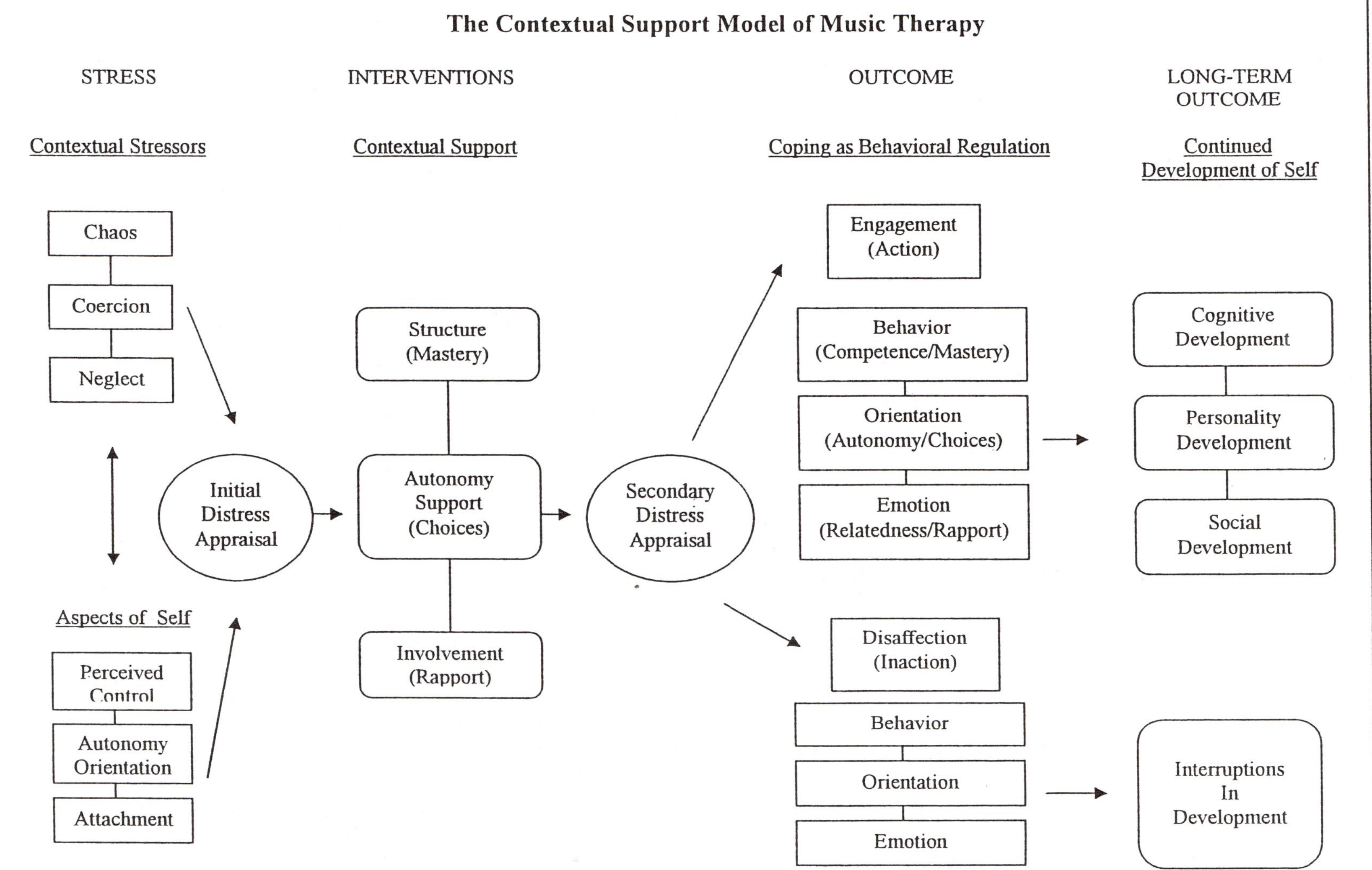

Figure 1. A Contextual Support Model of Music Therapy

1. *Contextual Stressor.* The hospital environment is defined as an objectively stressful environment. Characteristics of the hospital environment that threaten children's basic psychological needs for competence, autonomy, and relatedness are summarized under the rubrics of chaos, coercion, and neglect.
2. *Personal Attributes.* Children's age, cognitive development, social development, and self system processes interact with the objective stressor. This interaction influences the child's appraisal of the objectively stressful situation.
3. *Contextual Support Intervention.* Music therapy interventions alter hospital environments through manipulation of the social context (e.g., structure, autonomy support, and involvement). Music functions as a motivator, actively engaging children in their environment. Once children are engaged, the music functions to elicit and reinforce children's independent and purposeful actions. These independent actions can take the form of choice making, initiating changes in the current activity, initiating conversations, and experimentation with play materials. The resulting engagement may result in a secondary distress appraisal that differs from the initial appraisal.
4. *Outcome.* Based on the previous definition of coping, children's responses to the environment are measured as engagement or disaffection with the environment. Self-regulated behaviors are further delineated under the domains of behavior, orientation, and emotion.
5. *Long-term Outcome.* Long-term outcomes include continued and normative cognitive, personality, and social development. Failure to reengage with the environment may temporarily halt or interrupt development. Engagement also serves to influence continued development of self system processes.

This theoretical model proposes that music interventions can effectively create a contextually supportive environment, thereby increasing active coping behaviors. Recent research, investigating interventions designed according to the contextual support model of music therapy, documented significant outcomes for both environmental support and behavioral outcomes for hospitalized children (Robb, 2000). In order to more fully understand how music can provide contextual support during times of stress, it is important to define the attributes of supportive and stressful environments.

CONTEXT: ATTRIBUTES OF STRESSFUL AND SUPPORTIVE ENVIRONMENTS

Motivational theorists have argued that humans have fundamental psychological needs for competence, autonomy, and relatedness to others. These drives are easily seen in children. For example, the toddler who insists, "No, I do it" as he struggles to complete a task and then exclaims, "I did it!" upon success is demonstrating drives for autonomy and competence. The drive for relatedness can be seen in the child who clings to his mother when entering a new play group, looking for support and confirmation that the situation is safe.

In their 1994 motivational theory of coping, Skinner and Wellborn argued that children experience distress when they perceive threats to their psychological needs for competence, autonomy, and relatedness. Aspects of the environment can either support or threaten these psychological needs, thus contributing to children's stress appraisals. Chaos, coercion, and neglect are dimensions of universal stress that characterize stressful environments. In opposition are structure, autonomy support, and involvement, which characterize supportive environments.

Chaos Versus Structure

The first element of contextual support, structure, refers to environments that communicate clear expectations and consequences, provide optimal challenges, and provide positive feedback regarding competence. In contrast, chaotic environments are inconsistent, unfamiliar, unpredictable, and fail to challenge individuals to act. Hospitalization can be a chaotic experience for children. Hospital environments are often inconsistent, unfamiliar, unpredictable, and fail to challenge individuals to act (Bossert, 1994; Siegel & Hudson, 1992; Skinner & Wellborn, 1994). Chaotic environments challenge a child's sense of competence or control. Loss of control, a commonly cited source of distress, can lead to feelings of helplessness and hopelessness (Bossert, 1994; Gochman, 1988; Kellerman, Zeltzer, Ellenberg, Dash, & Rigler, 1980; Lazarus & Folkman, 1984; Melamed, 1991; Nannis et al., 1982; Poster, 1983; Skinner, 1995; Steward, O'Connor, Acredolo, & Steward, 1996; Trad, 1989; Worchel, Copeland, & Barker, 1987). Researchers emphasize a sense of control as necessary for positive mental health and a child's developing sense of competence. Feelings of control or competence are derived from experiences where children successfully master aspects of their environment. When environments are unpredictable and fail to communicate clear expectations, children's coping abilities are hampered (Ferguson, 1984). As a result, children may withdraw from or rebel against chaotic environments (Patrick, Skinner, & Connell, 1993; Poster, 1983; Skinner, 1995; Skinner & Wellborn, 1994; Worchel et al., 1987; Zeltzer, 1994).

Structure serves to diminish the effects of chaotic environments by encouraging children to be active agents in their environment. Music provides order and predictability, fostering feelings of security in children. This security enables children to reengage with their environment during times of distress. Music therapists reference three aspects of music interventions that create safe, predictable environments where children can master their fears and experience success: the natural structure of music, the ordering of session activities, and the client–therapist relationship (see Table 1) (Aldridge, 1993; Bailey, 1984; Barrickman, 1989; Brodsky, 1989; Christenberry, 1979; Fagen, 1982; Froehlich, 1996; Gettel, 1985; Hartley, 1989; Kallay, 1997; McDonnell, 1983, 1984; Micci, 1984; Osborn, 1997; Pfaff, Smith, & Gowan, 1989; Sims & Burdett, 1996; Turry, 1997).

Structure and order inherent in music is one of its most valuable attributes as a therapeutic medium (Clair, 1996; Gaston, 1968; Sears, 1968; Thaut, 2002a). Rhythm provides order in music, regulating sounds and silences across time (Radocy & Boyle, 1997). Detached and percussive sounds tend to stimulate an active response, whereas nonpercussive, legato music is associated with a calm response (Clair, 1996; Radocy & Boyle, 1997). Other musical attributes including pitch, melody, harmony, texture, and timbre also contribute to the listeners experience (Clair, 1996; Radocy & Boyle, 1997). While these are typical responses, musical experiences are unique for each individual. Idiosyncratic responses to music include behavioral (e.g., physical action), physiological (e.g., heart rate, respiration rate, blood pressure), and emotional reactions (Hodges,

1996; Radocy & Boyle, 1997; Thaut, 2002a). These emotional and physiological reactions to music are influenced by expectations of the listener.

Early and ongoing experiences with music of one's culture leads to musical expectations. Music in essence becomes predictable. This predictability is one reason people find comfort and reassurance in familiar music that it is predictable (Clair, 1996; Gfeller, 2002b). In chaotic environments, the structure inherent in music provides order and respite for young children. Familiar music, fingerplays, and participation in instrumental play represent normal childhood activities. Introducing familiar activities into stressful environments promotes feelings of comfort and security, which functions to diminish state anxiety and promotes active exploration and engagement with the environment. Flexibility, another characteristic of music, enables the therapist to modify musical elements to match the activity level and mood of hospitalized children, gradually leading them to greater engagement with their environment (see Table 1).

Table 1
Contextual Support Element: Structure

Source	**Characteristics**
Music	• Familiar music to create comfort and security; encourage action • Musical elements structure children's participation and responses • Musical elements to energize and motivate action • Flexibility of musical structure to facilitate independent and successful experiences
Session Format	• Repetition to create familiarity and predictability • Clear delineation of opening and closing • Challenge child at an appropriate level • Structure success experiences
Client–Therapist Relationship	• Monitor children's abilities and activity level to ensure successful experiences where children can master the environment • Provide children with positive reinforcement • Therapist becomes a familiar and supportive figure that encourages children to act on their environment

Note. Structure refers to environments that communicate clear expectations and consequences, provide optimal challenges, and provide positive feedback regarding competence (Connell & Wellborn, 1991; Skinner & Wellborn, 1994).

Coercion Versus Autonomy Support

Autonomy support, the second contextual element, encourages freedom of expression by permitting children to make choices and decisions about activities. In comparison, coercive environments provide few choices and constrain or control children's activities. Coercive environments provide few choices and constrain or control children's activities (Skinner & Wellborn, 1994). Enforced bed rest, restricted visitation, limited choices regarding daily activities and medical treatment, and expectations for compliance are common coercive characteristics of hospitalization (Bossert, 1994; Friedman & Mulhern, 1991; Poster, 1983; Sanger, Copeland, & Davidson, 1991; Siegel & Hudson, 1992). Coercive environments threaten a child's developing sense of independence and autonomy. Patrick, Skinner, and Connell (1993) describe autonomy as the connection between volition and action. Autonomous behavior occurs when children feel free to make and act on their decisions. Compliance and defiance represent nonautonomous behavior since both are reactions to another person's agenda. When children's activities and choice making opportunities are limited, their developing sense of independence and self-confidence may stagnate (Beck & Smith, 1988; Patrick et al., 1993; Skinner, 1995). Behavioral reactions to lost autonomy include boredom, depression, withdrawal, dependence, or defiance (Patrick et al., 1993; Poster, 1983; Skinner, 1995; Skinner & Wellborn, 1994).

Autonomy support encourages freedom of expression by permitting children to make choices and decisions about activities. Affording children opportunities to make choices and be independent are discussed in pediatric music therapy literature (Aldridge, 1993; Barrickman, 1989; Bishop, Christenberry, Robb, & Rudenberg, 1996; Froehlich, 1996; Kneisley, 1996; Magill, Coyle, Handzo, & Loscalzo, 1997; McDonnell, 1984). The flexibility of musical structures allows children creative independence through improvisation and song writing. Children experience creative freedom as they determine the tempo, dynamics, rhythmic structure, and form of their musical creations. Presentation of various musical instruments and materials also afford children opportunities to make choices (see Table 2).

Neglect Versus Involvement

Involvement, the third contextual element, is defined as a person's expression of interest, enjoyment, and genuine acceptance of a child. Involved adults are emotionally available and attend to the needs and interests of children (Connell & Wellborn, 1991; Skinner & Wellborn, 1994). Neglect, as a category of environmental stress, refers to the absence or diminished availability of emotional support in a child's environment (Skinner & Wellborn, 1994). Parental separation, increased parental distress, and sudden dependence on strangers to meet physical and emotional needs are aspects of hospitalization categorized as neglectful (Bossert, 1994; Friedman & Mulhern, 1991; McClowry & McCLeod, 1990; Melamed & Ridley-Johnson, 1988; Poster, 1983; Sanger et al., 1991; Siegel & Hudson, 1992; Trad, 1989). Children, especially infants and young children, look to their caregiver for emotional support during stressful life events. When emotional support is absent, diminished, or sporadic children will manifest anxiety through a variety of behaviors including protest, defiance, apathy, or withdrawal (Bonn, 1994; Carton & Nowicki, 1996; Holden, 1995; Melamed & Siegel, 1985; Poster, 1983; Skinner, 1995; Skinner & Wellborn, 1994; Zuckerberg, 1994).

Expression of interest, enjoyment, and genuine acceptance of a child defines the third contextual support element, involvement. Contextual involvement serves to mitigate the effects of a neglectful environment and builds a child's sense of security and self-worth (Connell & Wellborn, 1991). Because the music therapist's primary role is to emotionally support children

Table 2
Contextual Support Element: Autonomy Support

Source	Characteristics
Music	• Flexibility of musical structures allow for creative independence of children (e.g., improvisation) • Musical elements support children's participation; resulting security encourages musical exploration and independent responses
Session Format	• Children given multiple opportunities to choose instruments and materials • Children given opportunities to determine the direction of activities • Children given opportunities to contribute their ideas to the formation of a final musical product
Client–Therapist Relationship	• Independent decisions are encouraged and reinforced • Therapist labels the connection between children's decisions and their outcomes

Note. Autonomy Support encourages freedom of expression by permitting children to make choices and decisions about activities (Connell & Wellborn, 1991; Skinner & Wellborn, 1994).

and facilitate coping, they are able to devote their full attention to children's emotional needs, acknowledging their feelings and supporting them during times of distress.

Live music, by definition, involves the presence of another human. The music serves to create a supportive and familiar atmosphere, promoting interaction between children, family members, medical staff, and therapist (Bailey, 1983, 1984; Bishop et al., 1991; Lane, 1996; Marley, 1984; Turry, 1997). Structural elements, including rhythm and melodic contour, shape participatory responses. Turn taking, expression of feelings, and cooperative interactions are several participatory responses structured by music. Children also have extramusical associations. Lullabies associated with bedtime or one's mother is an example of an association. Perception of patterns within music and extramusical associations, can induce arousal and affective responses (Thaut, 2002a). These affective responses include physiological reactions and changes in mood (Radocy & Boyle, 1997). Music, therefore, can be used to promote interaction and create an emotionally positive environment for children and their families (see Table 3).

PERSONAL ATTRIBUTES AND COPING: A DEVELOPMENTAL PERSPECTIVE

Children's interactions with the environment produce individual differences in belief's about competence, autonomy, and relatedness to others. Environments characterized by structure, autonomy support, and emotional support promote the development of positive belief systems. Chaotic, coercive, and neglectful environments are detrimental to the formation of healthy belief

Table 3
Contextual Support Element: Involvement

Source	Characteristics
Music	• Familiar music and active music-making affords a shared experience that facilitates rapport • Familiar and developmentally appropriate music creates an enjoyable, shared experience
Session Format	• Children's interests and needs are kept central to activity selection and direction of the session • A flexible format allows the therapist to meet children's changing needs
Client–Therapist Relationship	• Unconditional acceptance of children • Meeting children where they are in terms of active participation and disclosure • Express sincere interest in children • Provide high frequency of positive reinforcement • Actively listen and attend to children • Respect children's ideas and support their efforts to act

Note. Involvement is a person's expression of interest, enjoyment, and genuine acceptance of a child. The involved adult is emotionally available and attends to the needs and interests of the child (Connell & Wellborn, 1991; Skinner & Wellborn, 1994).

systems (Connell & Wellborn, 1991; Skinner, 1995; Skinner & Wellborn, 1994). Three belief systems, or self-system processes, influence how children appraise and cope with stressful experiences: perceived control, autonomy orientation, and attachment. Formation of self-system processes is a dynamic, developmental process. Developmental level, therefore, influences how children appraise stress (Connell & Wellborn, 1991; LaMontagne, 1983; Nowicki & Strickland, 1973; Skinner, 1995; Skinner & Wellborn, 1994).

Perceived Control

Beliefs about personal control develop as children interact with and attempt to master aspects of the environment. The term locus of control is a construct that stems from social learning theory (Gochman, 1988). Locus of control is defined as a person's beliefs regarding their ability to create desired outcomes or prevent undesired outcomes in the environment (Connell & Wellborn, 1991; Skinner, 1995; Skinner & Wellborn, 1994). Researchers speculate that control beliefs are related to cognitive development, and may play an important role in children's conceptions of illness (Sammons, 1988; Skinner, 1995; Skinner & Wellborn, 1994). Research also suggests that locus of control becomes more internal with age (Neuhauser, Amesterdam, Hines, & Steward, 1978; Nowicki & Strickland, 1973). Examination of Piaget's theory of cognitive development supports developmental theories of perceived control (Holden, 1995; O'Dougherty & Brown, 1990; Woolfolk, 1990).

Piaget's Stages of Cognitive Development

Formulating interventions to mitigate the affects of initial stress appraisal requires an understanding of cognitive development and its influence on children's perceptions of control and illness. Jean Piaget's theory of cognitive development (1963) consists of four stages: sensorimotor, birth to 24 months; preoperational, 24 months to 7 years; concrete operations, 7 to 11 years; and formal operations, 12 years and older. Several researchers use Piaget's stages of cognitive development to organize discussions about stress and coping responses of hospitalized children (Brown, O'Keeffe, Sanders, & Baker, 1986; Ferguson, 1984; Holden, 1995; O'Dougherty & Brown, 1990), and children's understanding of illness (Bibace & Walsh, 1980; Corbo-Richert, 1994; Holden, 1995; Perrin & Gerrity, 1981). A brief description of each developmental stage is followed by discussion regarding the relationship between developmental stage and perceptions of control and illness.

Infants, birth to 2 years, experience their world through involuntary and reflexive patterns of movement. During the sensorimotor period, infants strive to master two primary concepts: object permanence and cause-effect relationships. Object permanence, the understanding that objects still exist even when they are not seen, emerges around 8 months of age and continues to develop through age 2. Infants also begin to understand that events may be related in a cause and effect relationship. For example, infants soon learn that when they move their arm, a rattle shakes; or when they cry, their mother picks them up (Holden, 1995; O'Dougherty & Brown, 1990; Wicks-Nelson & Israel, 1997; Woolfolk, 1990).

Early cause and effect encounters mark a child's initial experience with control. Because infants are unable to understand reasons for pain or distress experiences, they rely on emotional support from their caregivers (Ferguson, 1984; O'Dougherty & Brown, 1990). The importance of attachment formation and parental support during hospitalization are addressed in the discussion on Erikson's stages of psychosocial development (see Table 4).

The second stage of cognitive development, the preoperational stage, has unique characteristics that fall into two categories: logic and perspective. Characteristic of the preoperational period, are the development of symbolic schemes. These symbolic schemes include representational play (pretend play or miming) and verbal language. As children progress through the preoperational period they develop an ability to think about objects in symbolic form; however, this ability is limited to one-way logic. Reversing the steps of a given task is difficult for children during this stage of development. This explains why abstract thought and principles of conservation are difficult for preschool children (Holden, 1995; Wicks-Nelson & Israel, 1997; Woolfolk, 1990).

Magical thinking, animism, and transductive reasoning serve as additional descriptors of the preoperational child's logic. First, magical thinking describes the preoperational child's belief that a person's wishes or thoughts can make things happen in the external world. Second, animism describes the child's tendency to attribute life and feelings to inanimate objects, believing them to be alive. Third, transductive reasoning refers to an immature form of cause and effect reasoning. During this process, a child having observed two phenomena to co-occur will relate them to each other in a cause and effect relationship. Formulating this relationship occurs regardless of the

Table 4
Developmental Summary: Infants and Toddlers

Jean Piaget's Stages of Cognitive Development		Erik Erikson's Stages of Psychosocial Development		
Sensorimotor Stage Ages 0–2 yrs.	• Begins to make use of imitation, memory, and thought • Begins to recognize that objects do not cease to exist when they are hidden • Moves from reflex actions to goal-directed activity	Trust vs. Mistrust	Infancy 0–1 yr.	• Infant's needs for nourishment, care, familiarity are met; parental responsiveness and consistency
		Autonomy vs. Shame and Doubt	Toddlers 1–2 yrs.	• Greater control of self in environment-self-feeding, toileting, dressing; parental reassurance availability, avoidance of overprotection

Coping Strategies		Music Therapy Strategies: Infants & Toddlers
Ages 0–2 yrs.	• Parental Attention and Affection. Child will cry, reach, or call out for parent • Defense Mechanisms Turn away from source of stress, close one's eyes, sleep, or cry	• Involve parents and siblings • Empower parents by giving them strategies and resources they can use with their child • Alleviate parental anxiety by providing them with resources • Facilitate interactions that maintain the parent–child bond • Use familiar, age-appropriate music and materials

practicality or reality of the relationship (Holden, 1995; Wicks-Nelson & Israel, 1997; Woolfolk, 1990).

A second feature of this stage, perspective, is characteristically egocentric. Children at this stage have difficulty considering more than one aspect of a situation at a given time. Perspective is limited to the child's own perception of how the world appears. Preoperational children see the world and the experiences of others from their own vantage point. This is not synonymous with selfishness, it simply means children often assume that everyone else shares their feelings, reactions, and perspectives (Holden, 1995; Wicks-Nelson & Israel, 1997; Woolfolk, 1990). In terms of perceived control, children see themselves as central to the events they encounter. This thinking, however, is not a mature form of internal control and can lead to deleterious perceptions regarding responsibility for illness.

Research literature describes the preschool child's view of medical procedures as hostile in intent. Young children fear body mutilation, physical threats to the body, and separation from their parents. Due to their magical thinking, preschool children often relate to procedures with fantasy and can misinterpret reasons for procedures (Corbo-Richert, 1994). Needles, rectal temperatures, and catheters are often viewed as an assault on the body. Considering their egocentric nature, it is easy to understand how preschool children can view these experiences as punishment and in turn feel responsible for their illness and the resulting treatment. Psychological upset experienced by young children in the hospital is often the direct result of this preoperational form of logic and perspective (see Table 5).

Children in the third stage of cognitive development, concrete operations, acquire more mature forms of logic and perspective. During this stage, children can attend to more than one dimension of a problem, solve "hands-on" or concrete problems in a logical fashion, classify and seriate information, and understand the concepts of conservation and reversibility. Abstract thought, however, is still difficult. The number of tasks children master increases as they mature cognitively. During this stage, children take pleasure in sticking with difficult tasks and mastering new skills (Holden, 1995; Wicks-Nelson & Israel, 1997; Woolfolk, 1990). This strong desire for achievement and initiative explains why children may fear being under another person's control (O'Dougherty & Brown, 1990).

Children in the concrete operations stage may still view hospitalization and medical treatment as a form of punishment. Medical professionals are viewed as powerful and children may become overly compliant to avoid further "punishment" (O'Dougherty & Brown, 1990). Although children are developing a sense of control, they may relinquish control or attempt to change the context of the problem in response to stress. During the later portion of concrete operations, children begin to learn new strategies that enable them to maintain a greater sense of control (see Table 6) (Skinner, 1995).

In the fourth stage of cognitive development, formal operations, adolescents can think hypothetically, consider alternatives, and analyze their own thinking (Holden, 1995; Wicks-Nelson & Israel, 1997; Woolfolk, 1990). The development of executive strategies allows older children to plan their course of action, act intentionally, strategize, problem solve, seek help, and engage in preventative planning (Skinner, 1995). These higher cognitive abilities enable adolescents to use cognitive coping strategies and develop an internal locus of control (see Table 7) (Brown et al., 1986; Ferguson, 1984; Holden, 1995; O'Dougherty & Brown, 1990; Skinner, 1995).

Table 5
Developmental Summary: Preschoolers

Jean Piaget's Stages of Cognitive Development		Erik Erikson's Stages of Psychosocial Development		
Preoperational Stage Ages 2–7 yrs.	• Gradual language development and ability to think in symbolic form • Able to think operations through logically in one direction • Has difficulties seeing another person's point of view	Initiative vs. Guilt	Early Childhood 2–6 yrs.	• Pursuing activity for its own sake; learning to accept without guilt that certain things are not allowed; imagination; play-acting adult roles

Coping Strategies		Music Therapy Strategies: Preschoolers
Ages 2–7 yrs.	• Increased verbal and receptive language skills, but aspects of logic and perspective often lead to misunderstandings about illness/treatments • Seek interpersonal support from family or trusted member of medical staff • Behavioral Coping Strategies: Distraction, behavioral reframing, avoidance, self-effacing behaviors, ventilating feelings • Seek information through active observation of environment	• Use familiar and age-appropriate music and materials • Give children an active role during interventions • Give children opportunities to exercise their developmental skills • Provide opportunities for choice and control • Afford success experiences in coping and every day skills to promote self-confidence and self-esteem • Promote independence

Table 6
Developmental Summary: School-Age Children

Jean Piaget's Stages of Cognitive Development		Erik Erikson's Stages of Psychosocial Development		
Concrete Operational Stage Ages 7–11 yrs.	• Ability to solve concrete (hands-on) problems in a logical fashion • Understands laws of conservation; able to classify and seriate • Understands reversibility	Industry vs. Inferiority	Elementary–Middle School 6–12 yrs.	• Discovers pleasure in perseverance and productivity; peer, school, and neighborhood interactions become increasingly important

Coping Strategies		Music Therapy Strategies: School-Age Children
School-Age Children	• Seeking support from family members or familiar persons • Countermeasures; Avoidance • Distraction • Inhibition of Action • Seek Information	• Encourage child to exercise developmental skills • Build on child's ability to use abstract thought and cognitive coping strategies (e.g., imagination and imagery; exercises or breathing structured by music) • Involve parents and siblings in interventions • Engage child in an ongoing project that promotes the acquisition of coping skills or self-expression (e.g., active music-making for pain management; song writing for self-expression)

Table 7
Developmental Summary: Adolescents

Jean Piaget's Stages of Cognitive Development		Erik Erikson's Stages of Psychosocial Development		
Formal Operational Stage Ages 11–15 yrs.	• Ability to solve abstract problems in a logical manner • Thinking becomes more scientific • Developing concerns about social issues and identity	Identity vs. Role Confusion	Adolescents	• Consciously searches for identity; search is built on outcomes of previous crises

Coping Strategies		Music Therapy Strategies: Adolescents
Adolescents	• Emotional support from family and friends • Still use behavioral strategies • Addition of cognitive strategies: positive self-talk, attention diversion, thought stopping, talking with someone, problem-solving	• Build on adolescent's advancing abilities in the area of abstract thinking and problem-solving (e.g., teaching music assisted relaxation techniques) • Support familial and peer relationships • Support and build on the adolescent's emerging interests and abilities (e.g., song writing, music listening, music and art, lyric analysis, video production as forms of self-expression and active engagement)

Autonomy Orientation and Attachment

Beliefs about autonomy orientation and attachment represent two additional beliefs systems important to the appraisal process. Autonomy orientation refers to individual's beliefs that they are free to choose a course of action. This orientation develops as children experience a growing sense of independence. Autonomy, characteristic of development in the toddler years, continues to evolve and culminates with individuation from family during the adolescent years (O'Dougherty & Brown, 1990; Woolfolk, 1990).

Secure attachments made during infancy provide a foundation for future relationships and children's growing sense of relatedness (Holden, 1990; Lazarus & Folkman, 1984; O'Dougherty & Brown, 1990; Skinner & Wellborn, 1994). Children continue to rely on the support of parents, friends, and family in later years. Perceptions regarding the availability of that support depend on interactions with people and the environment. Erikson's stages of psychosocial development and the role of parents during times of stress illustrate how beliefs about autonomy and familial support are formed during childhood.

Erikson's Stages of Psychosocial Development

Like Piaget, Erik Erikson's theory of psychosocial development (1963) provides structure for discussion regarding developmental factors that influence the appraisal process. Erikson's theory of psychosocial development has eight critical stages, each leading to a positive or negative outcome. Successful resolution of each crisis leads to the ability to cope with future crises (Goshman, 1981; Woolfolk, 1990). The final three stages of Erikson's theory apply to adulthood; therefore, this discussion focuses on stages one through five.

The first stage of psychosocial development is critical to the formation of attachment beliefs. During infancy, children encounter the basic conflict of trust versus mistrust. As infants learn that they are separate from the world around them, they discover whether or not they can depend on others to care for them. If caregivers consistently meet infant's needs and develop a close, nurturing relationship, the infant will develop trust. Positive and consistent contact between the parent and child are important during the first year of life to establish a healthy parent–child bond (Goshman, 1981; Holden, 1995; O'Dougherty & Brown, 1990; Woolfolk, 1990). This healthy interaction between parent and child is an important support mechanism. Related to the parent–child bond are two normative fears: separation and stranger anxiety. For young hospitalized children, separation anxiety and fear of strangers are heightened and warrant intervention (see Table 4) (Holden, 1995; O'Dougherty & Brown, 1990).

Autonomy versus shame and doubt, Erikson's second stage, signals initial development of self-control and confidence. This period of development, characterized by the emergence of independence, serves as a foundation for beliefs about autonomy. Children, ages 1 to 2, acquire developmental skills that enable them to do such tasks as feeding, dressing, and toileting. It is important that children be given opportunities to do more on their own as they are developing a sense of autonomy. Reassuring and confident attitudes reinforce children's efforts to master new skills. Children who are not encouraged may begin to doubt their abilities to manage tasks independently and lack self-confidence in later years (see Table 4) (Goshman, 1981; Holden, 1995; O'Dougherty & Brown, 1990; Woolfolk, 1990).

During this second stage of development, children demonstrate strong attachment to their caregiver and use social referencing as they explore their environment. Social referencing is a phenomenon most easily observed when young children are in novel situations. Children use their parent as a "secure base" as they explore their surroundings and establish their independence. In the novel hospital environment, the absence of a parent, lost opportunities to practice newly acquired skills and limited opportunities for independence contribute to children's distress. The result can be developmental regression and a diminished sense of self-esteem (O'Dougherty & Brown, 1990). Children who develop a secure sense of independence and attachment, however, are expected to appraise and react to stressful situations more positively than children with underdeveloped autonomy and attachment (see Table 4) (Patrick et al., 1993; Skinner & Wellborn, 1994).

Children approximately 2 to 6 years of age are in Erikson's third stage of psychosocial development. Initiative versus guilt describes the conflict of this developmental period. Children are active and in constant motion as they undertake, plan, and attack new tasks. With initiative, however, comes the realization that some activities are forbidden. Children experience conflict between what they want to do, and what should and should not be done. This marks the initial development of morals or a sense of right and wrong (see Table 5) (O'Dougherty & Brown, 1990; Woolfolk, 1990).

Play is an important form of initiative, and pretend play is common as children imagine themselves in various roles. Children are eager for responsibility, and it is important that they receive affirmation from adults regarding their contributions. If children are not given opportunities for independent learning, they may develop a sense of guilt and come to believe that what they want to do is wrong (Woolfolk, 1990). The desire for independent learning and initiative illustrate continued formation of autonomy. Secure attachment takes on new dimensions, as parents develop strategies to support their child's need for increased independence (see Table 5).

Industry versus inferiority is the conflict children encounter during Erikson's fourth stage of psychosocial development. Children around 6 to 12 years of age begin to see the relationship between perseverance and the pleasure experienced when completing a job. In addition to perseverance, children begin to socialize and interact with people outside the immediate family. School and neighborhood environments present new challenges that must be balanced with challenges in the home environment. The child's ability to move between these environments and cope with multiple challenges—academics, friends, activities—leads to a growing sense of competence and autonomy. If parents do not support these experiences, the child may experience feelings of inferiority (see Table 6) (O'Dougherty & Brown, 1990; Woolfolk, 1990).

Erikson's fifth stage, identity versus role confusion, is characterized by adolescent's struggle to establish their identity. Sense of self begins to form during infancy, but adolescence marks the first time individuals consciously explore their identity. Successful progression through the first four stages equips adolescents with a strong sense of autonomy and competence. A strong sense of autonomy helps adolescents assert their desire to make independent decisions about their life. The industry and initiative experienced in earlier years contributes to adolescent's beliefs about their ability to act on their environment (see Table 7) (O'Dougherty, 1990; Woolfolk, 1990).

Adolescents still find support in familial relationships, but peers play an increasingly important role. Security found in supportive familial relationships and support from peer groups characterizes attachment during adolescence. The desire to make independent decisions reflects change in beliefs about autonomy. During hospitalization, independence and availability of peer support are limited. Interventions that reinforce beliefs about individual abilities and available support encourage adolescents to approach stress proactively (see Table 7) (O'Daugherty & Brown, 1990; Woolfolk, 1990).

COPING STRATEGIES AND DEVELOPMENT: CHILDREN IN ACTION

Coping strategies employed by children are heavily influenced by cognitive and psychosocial development (McClowry & McCleod, 1990; Melamed, 1991; Ryan-Wegner, 1996). Successful coping is partially dependent on one's repertoire of coping strategies. Younger children lack the cognitive and emotional maturity of older children, therefore, they exhibit a decreased ability to generate and apply self-control strategies (Melamed & Ridley-Johnson, 1988). Pediatric coping research indicate that younger children use primarily behavioral strategies, use of cognitive strategies increases with age, and the number of strategies children use increases with age (Bossert, 1994; Brown et al., 1986; Corbo-Richert, Caty, & Barnes, 1993; Ryan-Wegner, 1996). Tables 4–7 list coping strategies used by children according to age. Notice the relationship between cognitive development, emotional development, and the coping strategies for each stage of development. Based on these three factors, the table recommends specific considerations for the music therapist.

Parental attention and affection are the most effective coping resource for infants and toddlers (Ferguson, 1984; Holden, 1995; O'Dougherty & Brown, 1990). Young children communicate their desire for emotional support by crying, reaching, or calling out for a parent. Defense mechanisms are another coping mechanism commonly used by infants and toddlers. Turning away from the source of stress, closing one's eyes, sleeping, and crying are examples of defense mechanisms used during times of distress (see Table 4) (Corbo-Richert, 1994; Ferguson, 1984).

Preschool children have the benefit of increased verbal and receptive communication skills, but aspects of their logic and perspective often lead to misunderstandings about illness and medical treatments. In a descriptive secondary analysis of research literature, Corbo-Richert et al. (1993) found that preschool children seek and accept help from others more than school age children do. Preschoolers, however, do not seek out as much information, nor do they engage in inhibition-of-action behaviors (remaining still for procedures). Preschool children tend to use the following behavioral strategies: distraction, behavioral reframing, avoidance, self-effacing behaviors, and ventilating feelings (Corbo-Richert et al., 1993; Ryan-Wegner, 1996). Preschool children may also cope by seeking interpersonal support from family or medical staff, or information through active observation of the environment (Ferguson, 1984). Given preschool children's tendency to engage in behavioral coping strategies, their limited abilities in abstract thought, and tendency to process life experiences through play; interventions that are concrete and active are warranted (see Table 5).

School-age children tend to ask more questions about their hospitalization and medical procedures and use more inhibition-of-action strategies than preschool children (Corbo-Richert et al., 1993). A study by Bossert (1994), revealed that countermeasures and seeking support were the coping behaviors used most frequently by hospitalized school-age children. Countermeasures are defined as physical and cognitive attempts to decrease stress by getting away from it or altering the effect of the situation. These results were congruent with Ryan's (1989) study of healthy school age children. Most frequently reported strategies in Ryan's study were avoidance and distraction. The second largest response category was seeking support. Although children are developing greater independence, Bossert (1994) and Ryan's (1989) research demonstrate that emotional support remains an important coping method for older children (see Table 6).

The coping behaviors of adolescents have greater breadth than those of younger children. Adolescents do not abandon behavioral coping strategies, but acquire additional strategies that are cognitively oriented. Brown et al. (1986) investigated cognitive strategies reported by children ages 8 to 18. Reported cognitive coping strategies included positive self-talk, attention diversion, thought stopping, talking with someone else, and problem solving. Reported use of these strategies increased with age for all categories. Despite increased use of cognitive strategies, adolescents still rely on emotional support from family and friends (see Table 7).

The preceding overview of coping strategies argues the necessity for interventions that promote active coping responses, especially in younger children. Music interventions provide children an active and developmentally appropriate means for self-expression, mastery, independence, and interaction in hospital environments (Aldridge, 1993; Bailey, 1983, 1984; Bishop et al., 1996; Froehlich, 1996; Turry, 1997). Consideration of environmental context and characteristics of the child enables the music therapist to design effective interventions.

COPING: THE ROLE OF ATTENTION AND EMOTION

In her book chapter, "Action Regulation, Coping, and Development," Skinner (1999) defines coping as action regulation under stress. When faced with stressful situations children will attempt to regulate their behavior in an effort to manage, resolve, or escape the source of stress. The role of the interventionist is to help children establish physiological, emotional, behavioral, and attentional states in which optimal self-regulation is possible. Skinner (1999) argues that when children are too upset, active, or distracted they cannot regulate their behavior in an optimal manner. The role of the therapists, therefore, is to inhibit actions that interfere with more effective self-regulation by using strategies that alter a child's emotional, physiological, behavioral, or attentional state.

Music-based interventions to promote coping in chronically ill children operate on this same principle. Contextually, the therapist uses music to increase the amount of structure, autonomy support, and relatedness that are present in the hospital environment. Additionally, music functions to modify a child's attentional focus, mood state, and arousal levels. It is hypothesized that by helping children to more effectively regulate their mood and arousal levels, they are able to become more actively engaged in their environment, exercise attentional control, and in turn experience more effective self-regulation. More than likely this is not a linear process. Questions remain concerning whether attention mediates changes in mood state/arousal levels, or whether mood state/arousal levels mediate changes in attentional control. In the section that follows, the author first summarizes portions of the biopsychological model of children's health presented by Compas and Boyer (2001), highlighting the relationship between attention and coping. Second, the author provides a brief overview of related research literature investigating relationships among music, mood, arousal, and attention—with resulting implications for future research and clinical practice.

Attention and Coping

Several authors have argued that attentional processes play a central role in how children appraise and respond to potentially stressful events (Beauchaine, 2001; Compas & Boyer, 2001; Wilson & Gottman, 1996). First, children must *orient* their attention toward a potential stressor. Second, children must *focus* their attention in an effort to appraise the situation as stressful or benign. In the event that the situation is deemed stressful, children must *shift* their attention away from the stressor and refocus on the identification and enactment of a specific coping strategy. Finally, the child must monitor changes in the stressor and the effectiveness of implemented coping strategies. Problems arise when children experience difficulty focusing and shifting their attention during times of stress. Compas and Boyer (2001) have identified three properties of attention that play a central role in how children respond to stress; these properties include attentional bias, attentional shift, and attentional focus.

Attentional Bias

The first step in the appraisal process is orienting to a particular stimulus in the environment. As humans we are unable to orient to and process all the information that is in our environment; rather, we must select what we will attend to at any given point in time. Given that attention is a selective process, it is important to give consideration to the role that attentional bias can play in stress appraisal. Compas and Boyer (2001) cite several studies that have found significant relationships between attentional bias and anxiety levels in children (Vasey, Daleiden, Williams, & Brown, 1995; Vasey, El-Hag, & Daleiden, 1996). In this area of research, investigators are interested in examining how a pre-existing condition will impact the type of information that children selectively attend to in their environment (Ehrenreich & Gross, 2002). For instance, children with anxiety disorders exhibited attentional biases toward anxiety-related and emotionally threatening stimuli when compared with their peers. Similar outcomes were found in a study where children and adolescents with posttraumatic stress disorder (PTSD) demonstrated attentional biases toward trauma-congruent information (Moradi, Taghavi, Heshat Doost, Yule, & Dalgleish, 1999). While much of the research on attentional bias has focused on children with clinical diagnoses such as anxiety disorders or PTSD, researchers are also taking an interest in how selective attention in nonclinical populations is affected during times of stress.

Wilson and Gottman (1996) called for an examination of relationships between attention, emotions, and motivation. Past emotional experiences, negative or positive, often influence how individuals direct their attention. For example, a child who has experienced difficulty with anesthesia induction during their first surgical experience often demonstrates a heightened sensitivity to negative attributes of the surgical experience upon subsequent admissions. The arrival of gowned personnel, preoperative medications, a stretcher, or anesthesia may well elicit memories of the past experience and result in combative or distressed behavior. In this scenario, the child's attention is focused on attributes of the environment that hold strong negative associations with the surgical experience. Thus, the child experiences difficulty orienting and refocusing his attention on the enactment of effective coping strategies.

Just as past experience can influence how we orient our attention, increased arousal or anxiety has been found to impact human performance on tasks that require focused attention. Wilson and Gottman (1996) pursue literature concerning the impact of arousal levels on human performance to explain this phenomenon. Easterbrook (1959) is credited with development of an "attentional narrowing" hypothesis. This hypothesis suggests that when an individual is engaged simultaneously in a primary and secondary task, that high levels of arousal should increase attention toward the primary task and diminish performance on the secondary task. Eysenck (1982), however, found that high arousal caused by incentives produced differential performance outcomes when compared with high arousal caused by anxiety. High arousal caused by incentives was associated with increased performance on the primary task, accompanied by no change in performance on the secondary task. In the case of high arousal caused by anxiety, performance was not affected on the primary task, but there was decreased performance on the secondary task. Wilson and Gottman (1996) argue that "attentional narrowing" does not adequately explain the effects of anxiety or heightened emotionality on performance. They argue that under conditions of high arousal caused by anxiety, there appears to be an expansion of attention to irrelevant cues, including negative self-evaluation and worry, which is likely the result of hypervigilance. Additionally, they note that there appears to be a decrease in attending to task-relevant cues.

This body of research suggests that children may experience an inability to filter irrelevant stimuli during times of high arousal, anxiety, or stress. When this occurs it takes all of the child's available attentional resources to execute a central task and they may experience difficulties in performing tasks that require divided attention. This body of research also suggests that when a person is motivated by positive incentives they experience improved performance. As clinicians, our goal is to help children better regulate their mood states and arousal levels so that they can focus their attention and engage in positive coping strategies. The use of music to directly influence and regulate mood states and arousal levels will be addressed later in the chapter.

Attentional Shift

One component of adaptive self-regulation is the capacity to allocate attentional resources among competing sources of information. Attention is a developmental skill with a substantial body of research literature dedicated to the subject (Cooley & Morris, 1990; Enns, Brodeur, & Trick, 1998; Plude, Enns, & Brodeur, 1994; Ruff, 1998). Although a thorough description of the developmental literature is beyond the scope of this chapter, it is important to acknowledge that as children's attentional skills develop they are able to exercise greater selectivity and speed in processing information (Cooley & Morris, 1990; Plude, Enns, & Brodeur, 1994). From a developmental perspective, it will be more difficult for a younger child to shift attention away from a negative or distressing stimulus such as pain. When attention remains focused on distressing attributes of a stimulus, the result is often increased negative emotional response and the exacerbation of symptom distress. Compas and Boyer (2001) note that children who are less able to shift their attention away from the source of stress may experience pain and distress more intensely and longer than children who can shift their attention more effectively.

Attentional Focus

The ability to focus or sustain attention on a given stimulus is also a developmental skill that becomes more refined with age. Researchers have found that children who can focus their attention more proficiently are better able to regulate their emotions and arousal (Balaban, Snideman, & Kagan, 1997; Gotlib & MacLeod, 1997). Compas and Boyer (2001) illustrate the connection between attentional focus and emotion referencing their work with children who have recurrent abdominal pain. The authors note that children who demonstrate a poor ability to regulate the focus of their attention may increase their focus on sensations of pain, thereby increasing their anxiety and fear, which in turn magnifies pain. Additionally, it is important to note that some coping strategies require more attentional resources than others. During times of great anxiety or distress, children may be unable to engage in strategies that make substantial demands on their attentional resources. For example, problem solving requires substantial attentional focus and may be less effectively used or inaccessible when attention is distracted or unavailable. It will be important for clinicians to assess a patient's attentional resources and select interventions accordingly. Clinically, one is also inclined to ask whether diminishing state anxiety frees up attentional resources. If so, it would appear prudent to use interventions that modify mood states and arousal levels such that patients are better able to regulate their attentional focus.

Music, Attention, Mood, and Arousal

The role that attention plays in the processes of appraisal and coping has important implications for interventionists. Compas and Boyer (2001) emphasize that enhancement of attentional control and the capacity to shift attention will likely enhance children's abilities to manage their pain and stress responses to illness. The question that remains is, how can interventionists directly impact children's attentional abilities during times of stress? Based on evidence that anxiety will impact a person's ability to shift and focus attention, it will be prudent to examine how reduction of state anxiety impacts a child's ability to selectively orient and remained focused on nonthreatening stimuli during times of stress. Refocusing attention on nonthreatening stimuli would be appropriate for younger children whose attentional abilities are less developed; however, this approach would also be appropriate for older children/adolescents during times of acute stress when attentional shift may be more difficult and attentional biases more pronounced. During times of prolonged stress, older children/adolescents would benefit from interventions that free up attentional resources for the purpose of problem-solving and considering alternative reactions to threatening stimuli (Compas & Boyer, 2001; Kindt, Brosschot, & Everaerd, 1997; Plude et al., 1994; Wilson & Gottman, 1996). There is already a substantial body of research establishing music as an effective medium for altering mood states and diminishing state anxiety (Abeles, 1980; Hodges, 1996; Husain, Thompson, & Schellenberg, 2002; Standley, 2000; Thaut, 2002a, 2002b). Whether or not music can effectively alter mood states and state anxiety to improve attentional skills in chronically ill children is an area of research that warrants further attention.

Arousal-Mood Hypothesis

Music perception research must be consulted as we begin to examine relationships among music, mood, arousal levels, and attention. The reader is referred to Hodges (1996) and Husain and colleagues (2002) for an extensive review of research documenting the impact of music on mood and arousal in the listener. Clearly, music has the ability to alter mood states and arousal levels in listeners; yet, if music-based interventions are to produce consistent and reliable treatment outcomes, research will need to isolate the variables responsible for mediating these changes.

Based on an extensive review of related research, Husain and colleagues (2002) propose an arousal-mood hypothesis. This hypothesis suggests that listening to music affects arousal and mood, which in turn influences performance on a variety of cognitive tasks. In their study, Husain and colleagues demonstrated that manipulations in musical tempo affected arousal but not mood in the listener, whereas manipulations of mode affected mood but not arousal. Additionally, the authors found that performance on a spatial task was enhanced when listeners were moderately aroused and in a pleasant mood state.

Husain and colleagues' (2002) proposal that improved cognitive performance is likely mediated by music's impact on arousal and mood has important implications for clinical research in the area coping and chronic illness. For example, initial studies that have examined the use of active music engagement to increase coping behaviors in young children have focused on the manipulation of environmental and musical attributes that promote competence, autonomy, and relatedness (Robb, 2000; Robb & Ebberts, 2003a, 2003b). These studies have documented that the music intervention possessed significantly higher levels of contextual support and that in the presence of this support patients demonstrated significantly more active coping behaviors. A current study, however, points to other attributes of music that may be equally responsible for eliciting higher levels of behavioral engagement in chronically ill children (Robb & Clair, in progress).

In this study, children are being randomly assigned to an active music condition, a music listening condition, or a control condition. The authors have observed an orienting response that occurs in both music conditions. During the music listening condition, when children hear a familiar piece of music they tend to orient to the source of the music and comment on its familiarity. This is generally followed by a change in their affective response and level of behavioral engagement with the music. Although levels of behavioral activation are higher in the active music condition, the initial orienting response is curious and raises questions about the underlying mechanisms responsible for changes observed in these studies. It would appear that music, which if familiar and holds positive associations for the child may be functioning to alter the child's mood state. These responses are consistent with a substantial body of research that has examined music as a mood induction technique (Hodges, 1996; Thaut, 2002b).

Numerous studies have documented the efficacy of music labeled as "happy" or "sad" to induce depressed and elated mood states in normal subjects, with music mood induction proving to be more efficient when compared with verbal induction methods (Albersnagel, 1988; Clark, 1983; Clark & Teasdale, 1985; Sutherland, Newman, & Rachman, 1982). Thaut (2002b) discusses the therapeutic relevance of *musical mood induction,* noting that this technique enables the therapist to access desired associative memory networks of the patient. For example, the systematic use of music to elevate a patient's mood may lead the patient to recall positive memories that break the cycle of negative or anxious thoughts that produce corresponding mood states. Musical mood induction literature and the associative network theory of memory and mood (Bower, 1981) would support the aforementioned arguments that music may be functioning to alter these pediatric patient's mood states making them more receptive to the music therapist's attempts to engage them in behavioral and/or cognitive coping strategies.

Husain and colleagues (2002) argue that mood and arousal represent different but real aspects of emotional responding. They note that mood state may have stronger consequences for cognitions (i.e., thinking and reasoning), while arousal may be more strongly related to activation or overt behavior. By altering mood states in a positive direction, the therapist may free up the patients' attentional resources so they can actively use the critical thinking skills necessary to problem-solve. Changes in arousal levels are equally important, as the level of behavioral activation often dictates the child's ability to manage their own behavior for the purpose of successful coping. A child who is hyperaroused will demonstrate difficulties remaining still for procedures or being able to orient his or her body toward a single stimulus. The hypoaroused child who withdraws from the environment for prolonged periods of time is at risk for developing depressive symptoms or developmental regression. In these situations, the music therapist uses principles of habituation and dishabituation to improve the child's ability to focus and sustain attention on a centralized activity. As the child's attention becomes more focused, they are better able to regulate their level of behavioral activation.

Habituation and Dishabituation

The principles of habituation and dishabituation are important to discuss when considering the role of music to sustain attention. In this case, music is being used clinically to orient children's attention toward a positive stimulus. As mentioned earlier, attentional focus may be difficult for younger children or for older children/adolescents who are experiencing high levels of distress. The music must orient the child's attention initially, but it must also function to sustain the child's attention over time.

Habituation to music occurs when a listener becomes inattentive to or unaware of the music stimulus in his environment. This phenomenon generally occurs when the music is monotonous and overly predictable, but can also occur when the music is too complex and unpredictable (Berlyne, 1971; Gfeller, 2002a). When music is to function as background for other activities, highly predictable and monotonous music that requires little attention may be desirable. If music is to be a focal point for attention, it will be important that the attributes of the music, including melody, harmony, dynamics, tonality, and rhythm, all function to sustain attention over time.

In his review of related literature, Huron (1992) discusses the "auditory orienting response." This response is described as an alignment of the listener's body toward the source of an unexpected sound. The orienting response can also include more subtle physiological changes in the listener (Rohrbaugh, 1984). Early work by Sokolov (1960, 1963) demonstrated that an auditory orienting response was dependent upon the degree of stimulus change. As a stimulus departs from the listener's expectations or habituated level, the probability of evoking an orienting response increases. In the case of music, changes in frequency, intensity, duration, and location of sound often produce orientation responses in the listener. Interestingly, Huron (1992) found that increases in stimulus level were more effective in evoking a neurological state of attentiveness than equivalent decreases in the music stimulus. For example, crescendos were more easily detected by the listener than diminuendos. Similarly, the additions of voices or instrumentation in a piece of music were more easily noticed than the subtraction of an equal number of voices or instruments.

The implication for the practicing music therapist is that once the patient is oriented to the music stimulus, maintenance of attentional focus will be dependent upon the systematic variation of the music stimulus. This means that the therapist must continually monitor the patient for signs of habituation to the music stimulus. If the patient begins to habituate to the stimulus, the therapist must change musical attributes of the piece or discontinue the music in order to sustain the child's engagement in a centralized activity. With young patients, this may require frequent shifts in music-based activities. The therapist must also monitor the patient for signs of overstimuluation. In her discussion of music, aesthetics, and therapy, Gfeller (2002a) argues that music is not inherently therapeutic. The simple introduction of music into an environment without careful assessment of the acoustical properties of the facility, age and musical preference of the listener, and attributes of the music that is selected for therapeutic purposes can have the unintended result of heightening anxiety and tension levels in the patient.

Using principles of habituation and dishabituation, the therapist adjusts musical stimuli to maintain optimal levels of arousal and focused attention in the patient. Injection of change through novel events within the music function to increase or recapture attention, whereas the maintenance of predictable and familiar music patterns function to diminish heightened levels of arousal in the listener. Hence, music is argued to be a viable tool for augmenting or diminishing arousal levels in patients during times of stress.

CONCLUSION

The goal of music-based interventions is not to change or teach self-regulatory skills in pediatric patients. It is very difficult to change already established forms of self-regulation that have been shaped over the years as the child or adolescent interacts within a variety of social contexts. In fact, efforts to teach new self-regulatory skills during times of stress will only place additional burdens on the child's capacity to self-regulate. Skinner (1999) argues that the focus needs to be on the construction and promotion of "adaptive action tendencies."

As discussed in this chapter, the therapist uses music to alter attributes of the environment. Specifically, the therapist modifies the environment so that patients experience increased opportunities to exercise their competence, autonomy, and relatedness with others while hospitalized. Structurally this is the first step, but the true mediating factor may lie with the use of music to impact mood states and arousal levels in children during times of stress. Changes in mood state and arousal level may prove to be the mechanisms by which children can become more actively engaged in their environment and in turn exercise more effective self-regulation. Additional research that directly examines relationships between mood, arousal levels, and music in pediatric patients with chronic illness will be necessary to increase our understanding of the specific mechanisms responsible for the positive clinical changes documented in pediatric patients. These are exciting times as we continue to build the scientific foundation for evidence-based practice in music therapy. Current and continued research efforts enable therapists to deliver the most efficacious treatment interventions for their patients and empower healthcare providers with information that will lead to the increased availability of music therapy services for pediatric patients and their families.

REFERENCES

Abeles, H. F. (1980). Responses to music. In D. A. Hodges (Ed.), *Handbook of music psychology* (pp. 105–140). Lawrence, KS: National Association for Music Therapy.

Ack, M. (1993). The psychological environment of a children's hospital. In M. C. Roberts, G. P. Koocher, D. K. Routh, & D. J. Willis (Eds.), *Readings in pediatric psychology* (pp. 33–39). New York: Plenum Press.

Albersnagel, F. A. (1988). Veltan and musical mood induction procedures: A comparison with accessibility of thought associations. *Behavior Research and Therapy, 26,* 79–96.

Aldridge, K. (1993). The use of music to relieve pre-operational anxiety in children attending day surgery. *The Australian Journal of Music Therapy, 4,* 19–35.

Bailey, L. M. (1983). The effects of live music versus tape-recorded music on hospitalized cancer patients. *Music Therapy, 3,* 17–28.

Bailey, L. M. (1984). The use of songs in music therapy with cancer patients and their families. *Music Therapy, 4,* 5–17.

Balaban, M. T., Snideman, N., & Kagan, J. (1997). Attention, emotion, and reactivity in infancy and early childhood. In P. J. Lang, R. F. Simons, & M. Balaban (Eds.), *Attention and orienting: Sensory and motivational processes* (pp. 369–391). New Jersey: Lawrence Erlbaum Associates.

Barrickman, J. (1989). A developmental music therapy approach for preschool hospitalized children. *Music Therapy, 7,* 10–17.

Beauchaine, T. (2001). Vagal tone, development, and Gray's motivational theory: Toward an integrated model of autonomic nervous system functioning in psychology. *Development and Psychopathology, 13,* 183–214.

Beck, S., & Smith, L. K. (1988). Personality and social skills assessment of children, with special reference to somatic disorders. In P. Karoly (Ed.), *Handbook of child health assessment* (pp.149–172). New York: John Wiley and Sons.

Berlyne, D. E. (1971). *Aesthetics and psychobiology*. New York: Appleton-Century-Crofts.

Bibace, R., & Walsh, M. (1980). Development of children's concepts of illness. *Pediatrics, 66,* 912–917.

Bishop, B., Christenberry, A., Robb, S., & Rudenberg, M. T. (1996). Music therapy and child life interventions with pediatric burn patients. In M. A. Froehlich (Ed.), *Music therapy with hospitalized children: A creative arts child life approach* (pp. 87–108). Cherry Hill, NJ: Jeffrey Books.

Bonn, M. (1994). The effects of hospitalization on children: A review. *Curationis, 17,* 20–24.

Bossert, E. (1994). Factors influencing the coping of hospitalized school-age children. *Journal of Pediatric Nursing, 9,* 299–306.

Bower, G. H. (1981). Mood and memory. *American Psychologist, 36,* 129–148.

Brodsky, W. (1989). Music therapy as an intervention for children with cancer in isolation rooms.

Music Therapy, 8, 17–34.

Broers, S., Hengeveld, M. W., Kaptein, A. A., Le Cessie, S., van de Loo F., & de Vries, T. (1998). Are pretransplant psychological variables related to survival after bone marrow transplantation? A prospective study of 123 consecutive patients. *Journal of Psychosomatic Research, 45,* 341–351.

Brown, J. M., O'Keeffe, J., Sanders, S. H., & Baker, B. (1986). Developmental changes in children's cognition to stressful and painful situations. *Journal of Pediatric Psychology, 11,* 343–357.

Carton, J. S., & Nowicki, S. (1996). Origins of generalized control expectancies: Reported child stress and observed maternal control and warmth. *The Journal of Social Psychology, 136,* 753–760.

Christenberry, E. (1979). The use of music therapy with burn patients. *Journal of Music Therapy, 16,* 138–148.

Clair, A. A. (1996). *Therapeutic uses of music with older adults.* Baltimore: Health Professions Press.

Clark, D. (1983). On the induction of depressed mood in the laboratory: Evaluation of the Velten and musical procedures. *Advances in Behavior Research and Therapy, 5,* 27–49.

Clark, D., & Teasdale, J. (1985). Constraints of the effects of mood on memory. *Journal of Personality and Social Psychology, 48,* 1595–1608.

Compas, B. E., & Boyer, M. C. (2001). Coping and attention: Implications for child health and pediatric conditions. *Developmental and Behavioral Pediatrics, 22,* 323–333.

Connell, J. P., & Wellborn, J. G. (1991). Competence, autonomy, and relatedness: A motivational analysis of self-system processes. In M. R. Gunnar & L. A. Sroufe (Eds.), *Self processes and development: The Minnesota Symposia on child development* (Vol. 23, pp. 43–77). Hillsdale, NJ: Lawrence Erlbaum.

Cooley, E. L., & Morris, R. D. (1990). Attention in children: A neuropsychologically based model for assessment. *Developmental Neuropsychology, 6,* 239–274.

Corbo-Richert, B. H. (1994). Coping behaviors of young children during chest tube procedures in the pediatric intensive care unit. *Maternal-Child Nursing Journal, 22,* 134–146.

Corbo-Richert, B. H., Caty, S., & Barnes, C. M. (1993). Coping behaviors of children hospitalized for cardiac surgery: A secondary analysis. *Maternal-Child Nursing Journal, 21,* 27–36.

Daveson, B. A. (2001). Music therapy and childhood cancer: Goals, methods, patient choice and control during diagnosis, intensive treatment, transplant, and palliative care. *Music Therapy Perspectives, 19,* 114–120.

Easterbrook, J. A. (1959). The effect of emotion on cue utilization and the organization of behavior. *Psychological Review, 66,* 183–201.

Edwards, J. (1998). Music therapy for children with severe burn injury. *Music Therapy Perspectives, 16,* 13–20.

Ehrenreich, J. T., & Gross, A. M. (2002). Biased attentional behavior in childhood anxiety a review of theory and current empirical investigation. *Clinical Psychology Review, 22,* 991–1008.

Enns, J. T., Brodeur, D. A., & Trick, L. M. (1998). Selective attention over the life span:

Behavioral measures. In J. E. Richards (Ed.), *Cognitive neuroscience of attention: A developmental perspective* (pp. 393–417). New Jersey: Lawrence Erlbaum.

Erikson, E. (1963). *Childhood and society.* New York: Norton.

Eysenck, M. W. (1982). *Attention and arousal: Cognition and performance.* New York: Springer-Verlag.

Fagen, T. S. (1982). Music therapy in the treatment of anxiety and fear in terminal pediatric patients. *Music Therapy, 2,* 13–23.

Ferguson, C. K. (1984). Childhood coping: Adaptive behavior during intensive care hospitalization. *Critical Care Quarterly,* 81–93.

Frank, N. C., Blount, R. L., & Brown, R. T. (1997). Attributions, coping, and adjustment in children with cancer. *Journal of Pediatric Psychology, 22,* 563–577.

Friedman, A. G., & Mulhern, R. K. (1991). Psychological adjustment among children who are long-term survivors of cancer. In J. H. Johnson & S. B. Johnson (Eds.), *Advances in Child Health Psychology* (pp. 16–27). Gainesville, FL: University of Florida Press.

Froehlich, M. A. (1984). A comparison of the effect of music therapy and medical play therapy on verbalization behavior of pediatric patients. *Journal of Music Therapy, 21,* 2–15.

Froehlich, M. A. (1996). *Music therapy with hospitalized children: A creative arts child life approach.* Cherry Hill, NJ: Jeffrey Books.

Gaston, E. T. (1968). Man and music. In E. T. Gaston (Ed.), *Music in therapy* (pp. 7–29). New York: Macmillan.

Gettel, M. (1985). *The use of song writing to reduce anxiety in children undergoing cardiac catheterization.* Unpublished master's thesis, Hahnemann University, Philadelphia, PA.

Gfeller, K. (2002a). The function of aesthetic stimuli in the therapeutic process. In R. G. Unkefer & M. H. Thaut (Eds.), *Music therapy in the treatment of adults with mental disorders: Theoretical bases and clinical interventions* (pp. 68–85). St. Louis: MMB Music.

Gfeller, K. (2002b). Music as communication. In R. G. Unkefer & M. H. Thaut (Eds.), *Music therapy in the treatment of adults with mental disorders: Theoretical bases and clinical interventions* (pp. 42–59). St. Louis: MMB Music.

Gochman, D. S. (1988). Assessing children's health concepts. In P. Karoly (Ed.), *Handbook of child health assessment* (pp. 332–356). New York: John Wiley & Sons.

Goshman, B. (1981). The hospitalized child and the need for mastery. *Issues in Comprehensive Pediatric Nursing, 5,* 67–76.

Gotlib, I., & MacLeod, C. (1997). Information processing in anxiety and depression: A cognitive-developmental perspective. In J. A. Burack & J. T. Enns (Eds.), *Attention, development, and psychopathology* (pp. 350–378). New York: Guilford Press.

Grootenhuis, M. A., & Last, B. F. (2001). Children with cancer with different survival perspectives: Defensiveness, control strategies, and psychological adjustment. *Psycho-Oncology, 10,* 305–314.

Hartley, K. E. (1989). *The effect of subject improvised recorded music on the stories of chronically ill latency aged children.* Unpublished master's thesis, Hahnemann University, Philadelphia, PA.

Hilliard, R. E. (2001). The effects of music therapy-based bereavement groups on mood and behavior of grieving children: A pilot study. *Journal of Music Therapy, 38,* 291–306.

Hodges, D. A. (Ed.). (1996). *Handbook of music psychology* (2nd ed.). San Antonio, TX: University of Texas at San Antonio IMR Press.

Holden, P. (1995). Psychosocial factors affecting a child's capacity to cope with surgery and recovery. *Seminars in Perioperative Nursing, 4,* 75–79.

Huron, D. (1992). The ramp archetype and the maintenance of passive auditory attention. *Music Perception, 10,* 83–92.

Husain, G., Thompson, W. F., & Schellenberg, E. G. (2002). Effects of musical tempo and mode on arousal, mood, and spatial abilities. *Music Perception, 20,* 151–171.

Jemal, A., Murray, T., Samuels, A., Ghafoor, A., Ward, E., & Thun, M. (2003). Cancer statistics, 2003. *CA: A Cancer Journal for Clinicians, 53,* 5–26.

Kallay, V. (1997). Music therapy applications in the pediatric medical setting: Child development, pain management, and choices. In J. Loewy (Ed.), *Music therapy and pediatric pain* (pp. 33–43). Cherry Hill, NJ: Jeffrey Books.

Kaplan, S. L., Busner, J., Weinhold, C., & Lenon, P. (1987). Depressive symptoms in children and adolescents with cancer: A longitudinal study. *Journal of the American Academy of Child & Adolescent Psychiatry, 26,* 782–787.

Kellerman, J., Zeltzer, L., Ellenberg, L., Dash, J., & Rigler, D. (1980). Psycholsocial effects of illness in adolescence. I. Anxiety, self-esteem, and perception of control. *Journal of Pediatrics, 97,* 126–131.

Kennelly, (2001). Music therapy in the bone marrow transplant unit: Providing emotional support during adolescence. *Music Therapy Perspectives, 19,* 104–108.

Kindt, M., Brosschot, J. F., & Everaerd, W. (1997). Cognitive processing bias of children in real life stress situation and a neutral situation. *Journal of Experimental Child Psychology, 64,* 79–97.

Kneisley, S. P. (1996). Therapeutic play in the hospital. In M. A. Froehlich (Ed.), *Music therapy with hospitalized children: A creative arts child life approach* (pp. 139–148). Cherry Hill, NJ: Jeffrey Books.

Koocher, G. P. (1986). Psychosocial issues during the acute treatment of pediatric cancer. *Cancer, 58,* 468–472.

Kusch, M., Labouvie, H., Ladisch, V., Fleischhack, G., & Bode, U. (2000). Structuring psychosocial care in pediatric oncology. *Patient Education and Counseling, 40,* 231–245.

LaMontagne, L. L. (1983). Children's locus of control beliefs as predictors of preoperative coping behavior. *Nursing Research, 33,* 76–85.

Lane, D. (1991). *The effect of a single music therapy session on hospitalized children as measured by salivary immunoglobulin A, speech pause time, and a patient opinion Likert scale.* Unpublished doctoral dissertation, Case Western Reserve University, Cleveland, OH.

Lane, D. (1996). Music therapy interventions with pediatric oncology patients. In M. A. Froelich (Ed.), *Music therapy with hospitalized children: A creative arts child life approach* (pp. 109–116). Cherry Hill, NJ: Jeffrey Books.

Lauria, M. M., Hockenberry-Eaton, M., Pawletko, T. M., & Mauer, A. M. (1996). Psychosocial protocol for childhood cancer. *Cancer, 78,* 1345–1356.

Lazarus, R. S., & Folkman, S. (1984). *Stress, appraisal, and coping.* New York: Springer.

Leitenberg, H., Greenwald, E., & Cado, S. (1992). A retrospective study of long-term methods of coping with having been sexually abused during childhood. *Child Abuse and Neglect, 16,* 399–407.

Lindsay, K. E. (1981). The value of music for hospitalized infants. *Journal of the Association for the Care of Children's Health, 9,* 104–107.

Loberiza F. R., Jr., Rizzo, J. D., Bredeson, C. N., Antin, J. H., Horowitz, M. M., Weeks, J. C., & Lee, S. J. (2002). Association of depressive syndrome and early deaths among patients after stem-cell transplantation for malignant diseases. *Journal of Clinical Oncology, 20,* 2118–2126.

Loewy, J. (1997). *Music therapy and pediatric pain.* Cherry Hill, NJ: Jeffrey Books.

Magill,L., Coyle, N., Handzo, G., & Loscalzo, M. (1997). Cancer and pain: A creative, multidisciplinary approach in working with patients and families. In J. Loewy (Ed.), *Music therapy and pediatric pain* (pp. 107–114). Cherry Hill, NJ: Jeffrey Books.

Malone, A. B. (1996). The effects of live music on the distress of pediatric patients receiving intravenous starts, venipunctures, injections, and heel sticks. *Journal of Music Therapy, 33,* 19–33.

Marley, L. S. (1984). The use of music with hospitalized infants and toddlers: A descriptive study. *Journal of Music Therapy, 21,* 126–132.

McClowry, S., & McCleod, S. M. (1990). The psychosocial responses of school-age children to hospitalization. *Children's Health Care, 19,* 155–161.

McDonnell, L. (1983). Meeting the psychosocial needs of hospitalized children. *Children's Health Care, 12,* 29–33.

McDonnell, L. (1984). Music therapy with trauma patients and their families on a pediatric services. *Music Therapy, 4,* 55–63.

Melamed, B. G. (1991). Stress and coping in pediatric psychology. In J. H. Johnson, & S. B. Johnson (Eds.), *Advances in Child Health Psychology* (pp. 3–15). Gainesville, FL: University of Florida Press.

Melamed, B. G., & Ridley-Johnson, R. (1988). Psychological preparation of families for hospitalization. *Developmental and Behavioral Pediatrics, 9,* 96–102.

Melamed, B. G., & Siegel, L. J. (1985). Children's reactions to medical stressors: An ecological approach to the study of anxiety. In A. H. Tuma & J. Maser (Eds.), *Anxiety and the anxiety disorders.* New York: Lawrence Erlbaum.

Micci, N. O. (1984). The use of music therapy with pediatric patients undergoing cardiac catheterization. *The Arts in Psychotherapy, 11,* 261–266.

Molassiotis, A., Van Den Akker, O. B. A., Milligan, D. W., & Goldman, J. M. (1997). Symptom distress, coping style and biological variables as predictors of survival after bone marrow transplantation. *Journal of Psychosomatic Research, 42,* 275–285.

Moradi, A. R., Taghavi, M. R., Heshat Doost, H. T., Yule, W., & Dalgleish, T. (1999). Performance of children and adolescents with PTSD on the Stroop colour-naming task. *Psychological Medicine, 29,* 415–419.

Nannis, E. D., Susman, E. J., Strope, B. E., Woodruff, P. J., Hersh, S. P., Levine, A. S., & Pizzo, P. A. (1982). Correlates of control in pediatric cancer patients and their families. *Journal of Pediatric Psychology, 7,* 75–84.

Neuhauser, C., Amesterdam, B., Hines, P., & Steward, M. (1978). Children's concepts of healing: Cognitive development and locus of control factors. *American Journal of Orhopsychiatry, 48,* 335–341.

Nowicki, S., & Strickland, B. R. (1973). A locus of control scale for children. *Journal of Consulting and Clinical Psychology, 40,* 148–154.

O'Dougherty, M., & Brown, R. R. (1990). The stress of childhood illness. In L. R. Arnold (Ed.), *Childhood stress* (pp. 326–349). New York: John Wiley & Sons.

Osborn, C. E. (1997). *The effects of brief pediatric music therapy interventions on the mood states of chronically ill hospitalized children.* Unpublished master's thesis, Allegheny University of the Health Sciences. Philadelphia, PA.

Patrick, B. C., Skinner, E. A., & Connell, J. P. (1993). What motivates children's behavior and emotion? Joint effects of perceived control and autonomy in the academic domain. *Journal of Personality and Social Psychology, 65,* 781–791.

Perrin, E. C. (1993). Children in hospitals. *Developmental and Behavioral Pediatrics, 14,* 50–52.

Perrin, E. C., & Gerrity, P. S. (1981). There's a demon in your belly: Children's understanding of illness. *Pediatrics, 67,* 841–849.

Pfaff, V. K., Smith, K. E., & Gowan, D. (1989). The effects of music-assisted relaxation on the distress of pediatric cancer patients undergoing bone marrow aspirations. *Children's Health Care, 18,* 232–235.

Piaget, J. (1963). *Origins of intelligence in children.* New York: Norton.

Plude, D. J., Enns, J. T., & Brodeur, D. (1994). The development of selective attention: A life-span overview. *Acta Psychologica, 86,* 227–272.

Poster, E. C. (1983). Stress immunization: Techniques to help children cope with hospitalization. *Maternal-Child Nursing Journal, 12,* 119–134.

Pratt, R. R. (1997). *Hospital arts: A sound approach.* St. Louis, MO: MMB Music.

Radocy, R., & Boyle, J. D. (1997). *Psychological foundations of musical behavior* (2nd ed.). Springfield, IL: Charles C. Thomas.

Robb, S. L. (1996). Techniques in song writing: Restoring emotional and physical well being in adolescents who have been traumatically injured. *Music Therapy Perspectives, 14,* 30–37.

Robb, S. L. (2000). The effect of therapeutic music interventions on the behavior of hospitalized children in isolation: Developing a contextual support model of music therapy. *Journal of Music Therapy, 37,* 118–146.

Robb, S. L. (2003). Designing music therapy interventions for hospitalized children and adolescents using a contextual support model of music therapy. *Music Therapy Perspectives, 21,* 27–40.

Robb, S. L., & Clair, A. A. (in progress). *The effect of active music therapy interventions on anxiety and coping behaviors of children with cancer: Client and family satisfaction.*

Robb, S. L., & Ebberts, A.G. (2003a). Songwriting and digital video production interventions for pediatric patients undergoing bone marrow transplantation Part I: An analysis of depression and anxiety levels according to phase of treatment. *Journal of Pediatric Oncology Nursing, 20,* 1–14.

Robb, S. L., & Ebberts, A. G. (2003b). Songwriting and digital video production interventions for pediatric patients undergoing bone marrow transplantation Part II: An analysis of patient-generated songs and patient perceptions regarding intervention efficacy. *Journal of Pediatric Oncology Nursing, 20,* 15–25.

Robertson, J. (1992). *A survey of the practice of music therapy in pediatric medical settings.* Unpublished master's thesis, Hahnemann University, Philadelphia, PA.

Rohrbaugh, J. W. (1984). The orienting reflex: Performance and central nervous system manifestations. In R. Parasuraman & D. Davies (Eds.), *Varieties of attention* (pp. 325–348). Orlando, FL: Academic Press.

Roth, S., & Newman, E. (1991). The process of coping with sexual trauma. *Journal of Traumatic Stress, 4,* 279–297.

Rourke, M. T., Stuber, M. L., Hobbie, W. L., & Kazak, A. E. (1999). Posttraumatic stress disorder: Understanding the psychosocial impact of surviving childhood cancer into young adulthood. *Journal of Pediatric Oncology Nursing, 16,* 126–135.

Rowland, J. (1990). Developmental stage and adaptation: Child and adolescent model. In J. C. Holland & J. H. Rowland (Eds.), *Handbook of psychooncology* (pp. 519–543). New York: Oxford University Press.

Rudenberg, M. T., & Royka, A. M. (1989). Promoting psychosocial adjustment in pediatric patients through music therapy and child life therapy. *Music Therapy Perspectives, 7,* 40–43.

Ruff, H. A. (1998). Summary and commentary. Selective attention: Its measurement in a developmental framework. In J. E. Richards (Ed.), *Cognitive neuroscience of attention: A developmental perspective* (pp. 419–425). New Jersey: Lawrence Erlbaum.

Ryan, N. (1989). Stress-coping strategies identified from school-age children's perspective. *Research in Nursing and Health, 12,* 111–122.

Ryan-Wegner, N. A. (1996). Children, coping, and the stress of illness: A synthesis of research. *Journal of the Society of Pediatric Nurses, 1,* 126–138.

Sammons, M. T. (1988). Pain assessment in children II: Understanding recurrent abdominal pain. In P. Karoly (Ed.), *Handbook of child health assessment* (pp. 87–409). New York: John Wiley & Sons.

Sanger, M. S., Copeland, D. R., & Davidson, E. R. (1991). Psychosocial adjustment among pediatric cancer patients: A multidimensional assessment. *Journal of Pediatric Psychology, 16,* 463–474.

Sears, W. (1968). Processes in music therapy. In E. T. Gaston (Ed.), *Music in therapy* (pp. 30–44). New York: Macmillan.

Siegel, L. J., & Hudson, B. O. (1992). Hospitalization and medical care of children. In C. E. Walker & M. C. Roberts (Eds.), *Handbook of clinical child psychology* (2nd ed., pp. 845–858). New York: John Wiley & Sons.

Sims, M. G., & Burdett, R. (1996). Music therapy and child life therapy: Reducing preoperative anxiety in pediatric renal transplant patients. In M. A. Froehlich (Ed.), *Music therapy with hospitalized children: A creative arts child life approach* (pp. 125–135). Cherry Hill, NJ: Jeffrey Books.

Skinner, E. A. (1995). *Perceived control, motivation, and coping.* Thousand Oaks, CA: Sage.

Skinner, E. A. (1999). Action regulation, coping, and development. In J. Brandstadter & R. M. Lerner (Eds.), *Action and self-development* (pp. 465–503). Thousand Oaks, CA: Sage.

Skinner, E. A., & Wellborn, J. G. (1994). Coping during childhood and adolescence: A motivational perspective. In D. L. Featherman, R. M. Lerner, & M. Perlmutter (Eds.), *Life-span development and behavior* (Vol. 12, pp. 91–133). Hillsdale, NJ: Lawrence Erlbaum.

Slivka, H. H., & Magill, L. (1986). The cojoint use of social work and music therapy in working with children of cancer patients. *Music Therapy, 6,* 30–40.

Sokolov, E. N. (1960). The neural model of the stimulus and the orienting reflex. *Problems in Psychology, 4,* 61–72.

Sokolov, E. N. (1963). *Perception and the conditioned reflex.* New York: Macmillan.

Standley, J. M. (2000). Music research in medical treatment. In *Effectiveness of music therapy procedures: Documentation of research and clinical practice* (3rd ed., pp. 1–64). Silver Spring, MD: American Music Therapy Association.

Standley, J. M., & Hanser, S. B. (1995). Music therapy research and applications in pediatric oncology treatment. *Journal of Pediatric Oncology, 12,* 3–8.

Standley, J. M., & Whipple, J. (2003). Music therapy with pediatric patients: A meta-analysis. In S. Robb (Ed.), *Music therapy in pediatric healthcare: Research and evidence-based practice* Silver Spring, MD: American Music Therapy Association.

Steward, M. S., O'Connor, J., Acredolo, C., & Steward, D. S. (1996). The trauma and memory of cancer treatment in children. In M. H. Bornstein, & J. L. Genevro (Eds.), *Child development and behavioral pediatrics* (pp. 105–128). New Jersey: Lawrence Erlbaum.

Stuber, M. L., Shemesh, E., & Saxe, G. N. (2003). Posttraumatic stress responses in children with life-threatening illnesses. *Child and Adolescent Psychiatric Clinics of North America, 12,* 195–209.

Sutherland, G., Newman, B., & Rachman, S. (1982). Experimental investigations of the relations between mood and intrusive, unwanted cognitions. *British Journal of Medical Psychology, 55,* 127–138.

Tebbi, C. K. (1993). Treatment compliance in childhood and adolescence. *Cancer, 71,* 3441–3449.

Thaut, M. (2002a). Neuropsychological processes in music perception and their relevance in music therapy. In R. F. Unkefer & M. H. Thaut (Eds.), *Music therapy in the treatment of adults with mental disorders: Theoretical bases and clinical interventions* (pp. 2–32). St. Louis: MMB Music.

Thaut, M. (2002b). Toward a cognition-affect model in neuropsychiatric music therapy. In R. F. Unkefer & M. H. Thaut (Eds.) *Music therapy in the treatment of adults with mental disorders: Theoretical bases and clinical interventions* (pp. 86–103). St. Louis: MMB Music.

Trad, P. V. (1989). Stress and child development. *Advances, 6,* 42–47.

Trask, P. C., Paterson, A. G., Trask, C. L., Bares, C. B., Birt, J., Maan, C. (2003). Parent and adolescent adjustment to pediatric cancer: Associations with coping, social support, and family function. *Journal of Pediatric Oncology Nursing, 20,* 36–47.

Tschuschke, V., Hertenstein, B., Arnold, R., Bunjes, D., & Denzinger, R. (2001). Associations between coping and survival time of adult leukemia patients receiving allogeneic bone marrow transplantation: Results of a prospective study. *Journal of Psychosomatic Research, 50,* 277–285.

Turry, A. E. (1997). The use of clinical improvisation to alleviate procedural distress in young children. In J. Loewy (Ed.), *Music therapy and pediatric pain* (pp. 89–96). Cherry Hill, NJ: Jeffrey Books.

Vasey, M. W., Daleiden, E. L., Williams, L. L., & Brown, L. M. (1995). Biased attention in childhood anxiety disorders: A preliminary study. *Journal of Abnormal Child Psychology, 23,* 267–279.

Vasey, M. W., El-Hag, N., & Daleiden, E. L. (1996). Anxiety and the processing of emotionally threatening stimuli: Distinctive patterns of selective attention among high- and low-test-anxious children. *Child Development, 67,* 1173–1185.

Whipple, J. (2000). The effect of parent training in music and multimodal stimulation on parent-neonate interactions in the neonatal intensive care unit. *Journal of Music Therapy, 37,* 250–268.

Wicks-Nelson, R., & Israel, A. C. (1997). *Behavior disorders of childhood.* New Jersey: Prentice Hall.

Wilson, B. J., & Gottman, J. M. (1996). Attention—The shuttle between emotion and cognition: Risk, resiliency, and physiological bases. In E. M. Heatherington & E. A. Blechman (Eds.), *Stress, coping, and resiliency in children and families* (pp. 189–228). New Jersey: Lawrence Erlbaum.

Woolfolk, A. E. (1990). *Educational psychology.* New Jersey: Prentice Hall.

Worchel, F. F., Copeland, D. R., & Barker, D. G. (1987). Control-related coping strategies in pediatric oncology patients. *Journal of Pediatric Psychology, 12,* 25–38.

Zebrack, B. J., & Chelser, M. A. (2002). Quality of life in childhood cancer survivors. *Psycho-Oncology, 11,* 132–141.

Zeltzer, L. (1994). Pain and symptom management. In D. J. Bearison & R. K. Mulhern (Eds.), *Pediatric psychooncology* (pp. 61–83). New York: Oxford University Press.

Zuckerberg, A. L. (1994). Perioperative approach to children. *Pediatric Anesthesia, 41,* 15–29.

SEVEN

ᔓ

Procedural Support: Music Therapy Assisted CT, EKG, EEG, X-ray, IV, Ventilator, and Emergency Services

Darcy DeLoach Walworth, M.M., MT-BC

SEVERAL PEDIATRIC PROCEDURES in the healthcare setting have historically required sedation for successful completion including intravenous (IV) starts, computed tomography (CT) scans, echocardiograms, magnetic resonance imaging (MRI) scans, electroencephalogram (EEG) tests, and x-rays. The use of live music therapy interventions have resulted in the elimination or reduction of sedation required during these procedures (Walworth, 2003). Areas currently receiving music therapy for procedural support at Tallahassee Memorial Hospital (TMH) include CT scan, EKG/echo, EEG, X-Ray, IV starts, ventilator extubation trials, and emergency services. Due to the noninvasive status of these procedures, patient preferred live music successfully functions as a distraction to lower anxiety, decrease noncompliant behavior, and/or as a catalyst to begin the sleep process for patients unable to sleep prior to or during a procedure.

THE NEED FOR SEDATION VERSUS MUSIC THERAPY

Many healthcare providers consider chloral hydrate to be the sedation drug of choice for pediatric patients requiring conscious sedation (Reynolds, 1996) and is the sedative most often used for pediatric noninvasive procedures at TMH. Side effects most commonly seen in pediatric patients receiving chloral hydrate include nausea, vomiting, stomach pain, mild respiratory depression, and hyperactivity (Greenberg, Faerber, & Aspinall, 1991; Greenberg, Faerber, Aspinall, & Adams, 1993; Ronchera et al., 1992; Sifton, 1998). However, more serious cases of adverse reactions in pediatric patients have been reported including seizures, respiratory failure requiring bag ventilation, laryngospasm, significant increases in middle ear pressure, and sinus arrhythmia (Abdul-Baqi, 1991; Biban, Baraldi, Pettennazzo, Filippone, & Zacchello, 1993;

Granoff, McDaniel, & Borkowf, 1971; Munoz et al., 1997; Sing, Erickson, Amitai, & Hryhorczuk, 1996).

In order to improve patient care, TMH implemented a hospital-wide initiative to decrease the amount of sedation administered to patients. The age range of patients appropriate for music therapy assisted procedures ranges from birth through adulthood. The primary reasons patients need sedation for noninvasive procedures includes increased patient anxiety about the procedure and/or noncompliance during the procedure.

Pediatric patients have been found to have high anxiety levels associated with various aspects of hospitalization (Chetta, 1981; Malone, 1996; Robb, Nichols, Rutan, Bishop, & Parker, 1995; Scheve, 2002). Needle sticks, reconstructive surgery after burns, and being in an unfamiliar environment have all been found to increase pediatric anxiety (Malone, 1996; Robb et al., 1995; Scheve, 2002). Prior negative medical experiences can also lead to increased anxiety during future interactions (Zeltzer & Feldman, 1999). Staff and parental behaviors including giving the child control by letting the child be in charge, criticism, apologizing, and parental anxiety all lead to increased anxiety for the pediatric patient (Blount, Davis, Powers, & Roberts, 1991; Frank, Blount, Smith, Manimala, & Martin, 1995). Distress behaviors related to increased anxiety in pediatric patients include crying, screaming, verbal resistance, and physical avoidance (Blount, Smith, & Frank, 1999). These noncompliant or combative behaviors make it difficult to complete medical procedures and can create a cycle of anxiety for parents, staff and patients.

In addition to anxiety and procedural noncompliance, the music therapist is also called upon to induce relaxation and sleep states, using music as a nonpharmacologic sedative. CT scans require that patients either be asleep or that they remain still to create a successful image. Many young children are unable to remain completely still due to fear of the unfamiliar environment. If any movement is detected during a scan, the image appears blurry and the scan must be repeated. This can lead to increased cost of procedure and fewer scans completed during a given time.

Music therapy staff members are available to provide live music interventions to eliminate the need for sedation due to anxiety, noncompliant behavior, or inability to sleep. Techniques used to eliminate the need for sedation vary according to the procedure and individualized needs of patients and their families. Interventions are modified to meet the unique needs of each patient; however, the underlying principles for the music intervention remain constant. These principles include: (a) the use of patient preferred music to diminish anxiety and elevate mood, (b) the isoprinciple to diminish arousal levels and induce a sleep state, and (c) principles of distraction to redirect attention during times of distress.

IMPORTANCE OF PATIENT PREFERRED LIVE MUSIC

Patient preferred live music has been used successfully to reduce anxiety, increase coping skills, and shorten length of stay for pediatric and adult patients in the hospital setting (Caine, 1991; Scheve, 2002; Standley, 1986; Winter, Paskin, & Baker, 1994). Forming a preference for certain styles of music or specific songs/artists is a complex process. Many variables have been researched to determine what factors are involved in the development of music preference. Increased repetition or exposure has been researched and found to influence music preference (Hargreaves, 1984; Stratton & Zalanowski, 1984; Thaut & Davis, 1993). People with formal music training respond differently to certain styles of music than people with no formal training (Brittin & Sheldon, 1995; Morrison & Yeh, 1999). The music people are exposed to in their cultural environment plays a large role in people's music preference development, reinforcing the findings of increased familiarity and preference for certain styles of music for children through adults (Morrison, 1998; Morrison & Yeh, 1999; Siebenaler, 1999).

LeBlanc (1982) developed a model of music preference formation explaining the changes people experience in music preference over time. The cycle of preference formation can involve different variables each time a preference decision is made. When a person hears music, the brain interprets the music as a stimulus. This input information goes through physiological enabling conditions, basic attention, and the listener's current affective state before reaching the personal characteristics of the listener. Based on all these variables, the listener can choose to like, dislike, or listen to the music more before deciding. If the listener does choose to like the music, repeated listening of the music and heightened attention to the music is likely to occur (LeBlanc, 1982). As demonstrated through this model, making a music preference decision is a complex and involved process that varies over time for each individual. Finding and using each patient's preferred musical genre or song is an important component of every music therapy interaction.

Several music therapy studies have investigated the use of live patient preferred music to manage pain and anxiety. Children having laceration repairs in the emergency room reported less pain when listening to their preferred music (Lutz, 1997). Similarly, less pain was experienced by children receiving hypodermic immunization injections who listened to their preferred music (Megel, Houser, & Gleaves, 1998). Patient preferred music was also found to decrease pain and distress behaviors for children on oncology and burn units who underwent painful procedures (Clinton, 1984; Pfaff, Smith, & Gowan, 1989; Schneider, 1982; Schur, 1986).

ISO-PRINCIPLE

The iso-principle was proposed by Altschuler (1948) and has been used therapeutically to alter patients' mood states and/or physiologic reactions to stimuli (Bradt, 2001). The iso-principle technique consists of matching live or recorded music to the patient's current anxiety or behavioral state, gradually changing the music to facilitate the desired change in patient behavior or mood state. For example, if a patient is exhibiting anxiety behaviors such as increased heart rate, breathing, and negative verbalizations, music with a faster tempo, louder volume, and engaging style would first be played. Gradually, the music is slowed down in tempo and decreased in volume until the patient exhibited decreased heart rate and breathing pattern.

The iso-principle with recorded music was used successfully by Rider (1985) to reduce pain and muscle tension for adult spinal cord injury patients. This technique with recorded music was also used to successfully decrease heart rates in adults by Biedermann (1991) and Saperston (1995). The benefit of using live music over recorded music is the ability of the music therapist to quickly change the music stimulus as the patient's needs change (Standley, 2000). Patients often demonstrate frequent fluctuation between calm and anxious behavior; when this occurs the therapist must be able to reflect those changes by changing the music's tempo, volume, and intensity. Several studies have demonstrated the successful application of live music using the iso-principle to decrease pain in pediatric postoperative orthopedic patients (Bradt, 2001) and to decrease anxiety for preoperative patients (Aldridge, 1993; Chetta, 1981; Scheve, 2002).

DISTRACTION

Music as distraction to reduce anxiety has been investigated and found to be effective in several pediatric healthcare settings (Chetta, 1981; Malone, 1996; Robb et al., 1995). Music has the ability to impact attention. When music is used as distraction the therapist helps patients redirect their attention away from a stressful medical procedures or stimulus, toward a nonthreatening music stimulus. By reorienting and sustaining the patient's attention on the music stimulus, the patient is less apt to experience a stress response during the medical procedure.

Several clinical research studies have investigated the use of live music to redirect attention for the purposes of pain and anxiety management. Malone (1996) used live music to distract pediatric patients receiving needle sticks which resulted in a significant decrease in crying and behavioral agitation. Live music was also successful in decreasing pain for an infant receiving debridement for Steven-Johnson Syndrome (Schieffelin, 1988). Significant changes in positive behavioral engagement and diminished anxiety have also been found in response to live, interactive music interventions for pediatric patients in protective isolation (Robb, 2000) and those on a general pediatric unit (Froehlich, 1984).

COST EFFECTIVE MUSIC THERAPY WITH ECHOCARDIOGRAMS

Music for procedural support at TMH has been most successful during echocardiograms/ electrocardiograms. There has been a 100% success rate in eliminating the need for sedation in pediatric patients receiving these procedures (Walworth, 2003). In addition to completely eliminating the need for patient sedation, music therapy has decreased procedure duration, resulting in more effective use of staff resources.

Prior to the implementation of music therapy for echocardiograms, approximately 70% of patients ages birth through 5 years old receiving the procedure required sedation. When sedating a patient, an anesthesiologist is paged and a room is occupied for the administration of the sedation and for the recovery period. Recent Joint Commission on Accreditation of Healthcare Organizations (JCAHO) sedation standards also require that a registered nurse be present the entire time a patient is sedated. When using sedation, the entire procedure will take an average of 2 hours. Music therapy interventions, however, have resulted in a 100% reduction in the need for sedation with the procedure being completed in 15 to 30 minutes. Given that no sedation is administered, the services of a registered nurse and anesthesiologist are not required, dramatically reducing the cost and the number off personnel required to complete the procedure. In addition, space needs are reduced as no room is occupied other than the lab where the ECG/EKG is administered. Music therapy as procedural support increases the efficiency of the procedure, freeing up more staff time and resources for use in other areas of the hospital.

The process of using music therapy in the echocardiogram lab employs the use of distraction techniques. Patients who receive music therapy for this procedure at TMH range in age from infant through 7 years old. Establishing rapport with the patient in the holding area before going to the procedure room generally results in a less traumatic transition for the patient and decreased anxiety about the procedure. Once in the procedure room, the music therapist engages the patient in live music interactions that distract the patient from the procedure and procedural instruments. Because young children have such a short attention span, the music therapist often has to change instruments, songs, and activities rapidly. It is not unusual for some patients to require a stimulus change every few seconds.

Sedation must be administered on an empty stomach. Most caregivers are instructed to bring infants to the procedure with an empty stomach in case the patient requires sedation to complete the procedure. If the infant's anxiety level is high at the beginning of the session and he/she is not fully responding to music therapy, the parents are given the option to feed their child and continue with music therapy or to have their child sedated for the procedure. To date, all parents have chosen to feed their infant and continue with music therapy. For all 104 cases, sedation was not required and the procedure was completed successfully.

MUSIC THERAPY ASSISTED COMPUTERIZED TOMOGRAPHY (CT) SCAN

Because patients are required to lie completely still for a CT scan image to be captured successfully, pediatric patients are generally required to be asleep for the duration of the procedure. Despite sleep deprivation, pediatric patients often have difficulty falling asleep in an unfamiliar, noisy, and brightly lit environment, such as a hospital waiting area. If increased patient anxiety interferes with falling asleep, the music therapy staff member acts as the patient advocate in this situation by assessing environmental, emotional, and physiological variables that may be contributing to this problem, and offers suggestions. Environmental variables include the number of people in the waiting room and the activity/noise level in each room and hallway. Emotional variables include previous experiences with medical procedures that were negative and the quality of family support. Physiological variables include the patient's age and amount of sleep deprivation, if any. When a patient requires an IV for the CT scan, the increased anxiety due to anticipation of pain also becomes a factor for the music therapist to consider. Given that no two patients are the same, the music therapist must exercise fine-tuned assessment skills for the purpose of identifying and implementing music-based strategies that will meet the idiosyncratic needs of each patient and family.

The ideal music therapy assisted CT scan is quick and easy for the patient, family members, and staff. Each caregiver is instructed to sleep deprive the patient before arriving at the hospital. If this has occurred, the pediatric patient will usually be somewhat irritable and tired. The patient is then taken into a waiting room where lights can be dimmed or turned off and the child can be rocked or soothed by the caregiver while the music therapist provides live music. Live music traditionally consists of guitar and singing, although a music therapist is not limited to the sole use of these instruments. As mentioned earlier, the primary technique used is the iso-principle. Many times the patient participates in the beginning of the session by playing rhythm instruments and singing along, and during the session, the music tempo and volume gradually decreases to lower the patient's energy and anxiety level. Once the lights are dimmed and the patient is being rocked or soothed, a warmed blanket is given to wrap the patient, which will then be used on the CT scan table. If a patient is sleep deprived and has positive family support, the process generally takes about 15 minutes.

As mentioned earlier, unique variations in environmental, emotional, and physiological variables for each patient will sometimes requires a greater length of time to induce a sleeping state in pediatric patients prior to their scan. Once the patient is sleeping soundly, the music therapist then follows the patient into the CT scan room and continues playing live music as the scan is in process. Sometimes the patient will awaken during the procedure and be frightened due to the unfamiliar environment. When the patient hears the familiar music, usually the patient will fall back asleep and the scan is completed successfully. Once the scan is completed without sedation, the patient and family are able to leave, and the whole process from check-in to discharge is generally less then an hour.

Initial program data at TMH indicates an 82% success rate for music therapy assisted CT scans that are completed without the need for sedation. For 6% of the unsuccessful cases, the patient was not sleep deprived and received an IV just before the procedure. An additional 3% of the unsuccessful cases included patients who were not sleep deprived and family support was absent. Another 3% received an IV for the procedure and had to wait for more than an hour for the CT scan. The remaining 3% of unsuccessful cases experienced an invasive procedure that included needle insertion into a mass during the scan as well as IV placement.

If a patient is not sleeping soundly enough when transferred to the table, sometimes he/she is taken back to the waiting room or to the adjoining CT scan room to be put back to sleep before returning to the table for scan completion. Because caregivers are instructed to not feed their child in case sedation will be administered, infant patients often miss a feeding prior to the procedure which can prohibit sound sleeping. The initial trial for assisting the child in sleeping is always done without feeding first. If the patient cannot sleep soundly, the caregivers are given the option to feed their infant and then continue the scan, or sedate the patient before continuing. A majority of parents choose to feed the patient and continue with music therapy services, knowing that if for some reason the patient is unable to complete the procedure without sedation, the procedure will have to be rescheduled. At present, TMH has experienced 100% success in completing music therapy assisted CT scans after caregivers choose the feeding option.

MUSIC THERAPY ASSISTED ELECTROENCEPHALOGRAM

Electroencephalogram (EEG) patients are often required to be asleep during administration of the test. In addition to the anxiety producing variables mentioned in the previous section, pediatric patients receiving an EEG may also experience increased anxiety from the leads placed on the head. Occasionally, patients completing this procedure are given a mild sedative and have an adverse reaction to the sedation. In this situation, music therapy services assist in relaxing the patient enough to physiologically allow the sedation to take effect so the patient can fall asleep. The implementation of music therapy during EEGs has also resulted in reduced amounts of sedation required for patients to fall asleep. Procedures used during music therapy assisted EEGs are similar to those previously described for CT scans; again, the music stimulus is adjusted to meet the individualized needs of patients and families using the iso-principle.

MUSIC THERAPY ASSISTED X-RAY, IV START, AND VENTILATOR EXTUBATION TRIALS

X-rays, IV starts, and ventilator extubation trials are often anxiety-producing for children when they are unable to shift their attention away from stressful events and toward a nonthreatening stimulus. In these situations, music is used to reduce patient anxiety by redirecting the patient's attention toward a music stimulus and ultimately successful completion of the procedure. Each of these procedures is completed while the patient is awake and fully conscious, and therefore the patient can attend to whatever live music stimulus is present. Live music has been effectively used to decrease pediatric patient anxiety across a variety of situations (Chetta, 1981; Malone, 1996; Robb et al., 1995). The therapist plays live music that is familiar and preferred by the patient. As the therapist engages the child in music, he/she must continually assess environmental, emotional, and physiological factors that may contribute to the child's anxiety level, modifying the music stimulus to meet the child's changing needs.

NOTIFYING A MUSIC THERAPIST FOR PROCEDURAL SUPPORT

Music therapy referrals and notifications for procedural support at TMH vary from unit to unit. The CT scan area schedules outpatients and notifies the music therapy department in advance due to the early morning time slot usually used for pediatric cases. The echocardiogram area also schedules outpatients in advance and then pages the on-call music therapist once the patient is ready for the procedure. Any inpatient needing procedural support including IV starts, EEGs, X-rays, CT scans, or echocardiograms is able to notify the music therapy department the day of the procedure or by paging the on-call music therapist for immediate assistance. Finding out what referral/notification system works best for the music therapist and each unit will maximize the benefits of music therapy in each procedural support area.

REFERENCES

Abdul-Baqi, K. J. (1991). Chloral hydrate and middle ear pressure. *Journal of Laryngol Otolaryngology, 105,* 421–423.

Aldridge, K. (1993). The use of music to relieve pre-operational anxiety in children attending day surgery. *The Australian Journal of Music Therapy, 4,* 19–35.

Altschuler, I. M. (1948). A psychiatrist's experiences with music as a therapeutic agent. In D. Schullian & M. Shoen (Eds.), *Music and medicine* (pp. 226–281). New York: Henry Schuman.

Biban, P., Baraldi, E., Pettennazzo, A., Filippone, M., & Zacchello, F. (1993). Adverse effect of chloral hydrate in two young children with obstructive sleep apnea. *Pediatrics, 92,* 461–463.

Bierdermann, B. R. (1991). *Synchronization of a music pulse to listener heart rate: The effects of tempo changes.* Unpublished master's thesis, Temple University, Philadelphia.

Blount, R. L., Davis, N. J., Powers, S. W., & Roberts, M. C. (1991). The influence of environmental factors and coping style on children's coping and distress. *Clinical Psychology Review, 11,* 93–116.

Blount, R. L., Smith, A., & Frank, N. (1999). Preparation to undergo medical procedures. In A. J. Goreczny & M. Hersen (Eds.), *Handbook of pediatric and adolescent health psychology* (pp. 305–326). Needham Heights, MA: Allyn and Bacon.

Bradt, J. (2001). *The effects of music entrainment on postoperative pain perception in pediatric patients*. Unpublished doctoral dissertation, Temple University, Philadelphia.

Brittin, R. V. & Sheldon, D. A. (1995). Comparing continuous versus static measurements in music listeners' preferences. *Journal of Research in Music Education, 42,* 36–46.

Caine, J. (1991). The effects of music on the selected stress behaviors, weight, caloric and formula intake, and length of hospital stay of premature and low birth weight neonates in a newborn intensive care unit. *Journal of Music Therapy, 28*(4), 180–192.

Chetta, H. D. (1981). The effect of music and desensitization on preoperative anxiety in children. *Journal of Music Therapy, 18*(2), 74–87.

Clinton, P. K. (1984). *Music as a nursing intervention for children during painful procedures.* Unpublished master's thesis, The University of Iowa, Iowa City.

Frank, N. C., Blount, R. L., Smith, A. J., Manimala, M. R., & Martin, J. K. (1995). Parent and staff behavior, previous child medical experience, and maternal anxiety as they relate to child procedural distress and coping. *Journal of Pediatric Psychology, 20,* 277–290.

Froehlich, M. R. (1984). A comparison of the effect of music therapy and medical play therapy on the verbalization behavior of pediatric patients. *Journal of Music Therapy, 21*(1), 2–15.

Granoff, D. N., McDaniel, D. B., & Borkowf, S. P. (1971). Cardiorespiratory arrest following aspiration of chloral hydrates. *American Journal of Diseases of Children, 122,* 170.

Greenberg, S. B., Faerber, E. N., & Aspinall, C. L., & Adams, R. C. (1993). High-dose chloral hydrate sedation for children undergoing MR imaging: Safety and efficacy in relation to age. *American Journal of Roentgenology, 161,* 639–641.

Greenberg, S. B., Faerber, E. N., & Aspinall, C. L. (1991). High dose chloral hydrate sedation for children undergoing CT. *Journal of Computer Assisted Tomography, 15,* 467–469.

Hargreaves, D. J. (1984). The effects of repetition on liking of music. *Journal of Research in Music Education, 32*(1), 35–47.

LeBlanc, A. (1982). An interactive theory of music preference. *Journal of Music Therapy, 19*(1), 28–45.

Lutz, W. G. (1997). *The effect of music distraction on children's pain, fear, and behavior during laceration repairs.* Unpublished master's thesis, The University of Texas at Arlington.

Malone, A. B. (1996). The effects of live music on the distress of pediatric patients receiving intravenous starts, venipunctures, injections, and heel sticks. *Journal of Music Therapy, 33*(1), 19–33.

Megel, M. E., Houser, C. W., & Gleaves, L. S. (1998). Children's responses to immunizations: Lullabies as a distraction. *Issues in Comprehensive Pediatric Nursing, 21*(3), 129–145.

Morrison, S. J. (1998). A comparison of preference responses of White and African-American students to musical/visual stimuli. *Journal of Research in Music Education, 46,* 208–222.

Morrison, S. J., & Yeh, C. S. (1999). Preference responses and use of written descriptors among music and nonmusic majors in the United States, Hong Kong, and the People's Republic of China. *Journal of Research in Music Education, 47,* 5–17.

Munoz, M., Gomez, A., Soult, J. A., Marquez, C., Lopez-Castilla, J., Cervera, A., & Cano, M.

(1997). Seizures caused by chloral hydrate sedative doses [Letter]. *Journal of Pediatrics, 131*(5), 787–788.

Pfaff, V., Smith, K., & Gowan, D. (1989). The effects of music-assisted relaxation on the distress of pediatric cancer patients undergoing bone-marrow aspirations. *Children's Health Care, 18*(4), *232–236.*

Reynolds, J. E. F. (Ed.). (1996). *Martindale: The extra pharmacopoeia* (31st ed)., London, UK: The Pharmaceutical Press.

Rider, M. S. (1985). Entrainment mechanisms are involved in pain reduction, muscle relaxation, and music-mediated imagery. *Journal of Music Therapy, 22*(4), 183–192.

Robb, S. L. (2000). The effect of therapeutic music interventions on the behavior of hospitalized children in isolation: Developing a contextual support model of music therapy. *Journal of Music Therapy, 37*(2), 118–146.

Robb, S. L., Nichols, S. J., Rutan, R. L., Bishop, B. L., & Parker, J. C. (1995). The effects of music assisted relaxation on preoperative anxiety. *Journal of Music Therapy, 32*(1), 2–21.

Ronchera, C. L., Marti-Bonmati, L., Poyatos, C., Vilar, J., & Jimenez, N. (1992). Administration of oral chloral hydrate to pediatric patients undergoing magnetic resonance imaging. *Pharmaceutisch Weekblad: Scientific Edition, 14,* 349–352.

Saperston, B. (1995). The effects of consistent tempi and physiologically interactive tempi on heart rate and EMG response. In T. Wigram, B. Saperston, & R. West (Eds.), *The art & science of music therapy: A handbook* (pp. 55–82). Switzerland: Hardwood Academic.

Scheve, A. (2002). *The effect of music therapy intervention on pre-operative anxiety of pediatric patients as measured by self report.* Unpublished master's thesis. The Florida State University. Tallahassee.

Schieffelin, C. (1988, April). *A case study: Stevens-Johnson Syndrome.* Paper presented at the Annual Conference of the Southeastern Region of the National Association for Music Therapy, Tallahassee, FL.

Schneider, F. A. (1982). *Assessment and evaluation of audio-analgesic effects on the pain experience of acutely burned children during dressing changes.* Unpublished doctoral dissertation, University of Cincinnati, OH. (UMI No. 8228808)

Schur, J. M. (1986). *Alleviating behavioral distress with music or Lamaze pant-blow breathing in children undergoing bone marrow aspirations and lumbar punctures.* Unpublished doctoral dissertation, The University of Texas Health Science Center at Dallas.

Siebenaler, D. J. (1999). Student song preference in the elementary music class. *Journal of Research in Music Education, 47,* 213–223.

Sifton, D. W. (Ed.). (1998). *PDR(R) Generics™.* Montvale, NJ: Medical Economics Company.

Sing, K., Erickson, T., Amitai, Y., & Hryhorczuk, D. (1996). Chloral hydrate toxicity from oral and intravenous administration. *Journal of Toxicology-Clinical Toxicology, 34,* 101–106.

Standley, J. M. (1986). Music research in medical/dental treatment: A meta-dnalysis and clinical applications. *Journal of Music Therapy, 23*(2), 56–122.

Standley, J. M. (2000). Music research in medical treatment. In *Effectiveness of music therapy procedures: Documentation of research and clinical practice* (3rd ed., pp. 1–64). Silver Spring, MD: American Music Therapy Association.

Stratton, V. N. & Zalanowski, A. H. (1984). The relationship between music, degree of liking, and self reported relaxation. *Journal of Music Therapy, 21*(4). 184–182.

Thaut, M. H., & Davis, W. B. (1993). The influences of subject-selected versus experimenter-chosen music on affect, anxiety, and relaxation. *Journal of Music Therapy, 30*(4), 210–223.

Walworth, D. (2003). *Tallahassee Memorial HealthCare Music Therapy Annual Report.* Tallahassee, FL: Author.

Winter, M. J., Paskin, S., & Baker, T. (1994). Music reduces stress and anxiety of patients in the surgical holding area. *Journal of Post Anesthesia Nursing, 9*(6), 340–343.

Zeltzer, L., & Feldman, S. (1999). Soothing and chronic pain. In M. Lewis & D. Ramsey (Eds.), *Soothing and stress* (pp.195–277). Mahwah, NJ: Lawrence Erlbaum.

EIGHT

Music Assisted Surgery: Preoperative and Postoperative Interventions

Jennifer Jarred, M.M., MT-BC

THE USE OF MUSIC THERAPY INTERVENTIONS for pediatric surgical patients is steadily expanding in medical facilities. Although pediatric music therapy has been implemented for decades, pediatric surgical support was only first quantifiably researched about 20 years ago (Chetta, 1981). Most of the music therapy literature in the surgical arena has been conducted with adults, with more than 30 empirical research studies (Standley, 2000). Music was used as audioanalgesia for adults as early as 1914 in the operating room prior to anesthesia induction (Taylor, 1981). Researchers have measured the effects of music on both physiological responses such as heart rate, blood pressure, respiratory rate, mean arterial pressure, body temperature, hormonal levels and psychological responses such as state anxiety and stress levels in the pre- and perioperative periods (Kaempf & Amodei, 1989; Updike & Charles, 1987; Walters, 1996). Other researchers have tested the effect of music on the amount of anesthesia or pain medication required peri- and postoperatively (Allen et al., 2001; Nilsson, Rawal, Enqvist, & Unosson, 2003).

Standley's (2000) meta-analysis examined approximately 13 studies and revealed that music interventions beginning during the preoperative period yielded better results than when music began during the perioperative period. Significant results from various studies using music during the surgical experience include: reduction in preoperative anxiety (Sanderson, 1986), reduction in the amount of anesthesia required perioperatively (Lepage, Drolet, Girard, Grenier, & DeGayne, 2001), and reduction in pain or the amount of pain medication requested postoperatively (Byers & Smyth, 1997; Locsin, 1981; Nilsson et al., 2003). For an extensive listing of related research literature, the reader is referred to additional references provided at the end of this chapter.

Although the majority of adult surgical studies introduced music in the perioperative period, pediatric research reflects more emphasis on the pre- and postoperative periods. Favorable results from studies with adults lend to promising applications of music therapy interventions with pediatric surgical patients, although the interventions themselves may differ in nature. Listening to recorded music classified as "relaxing," "sedative," or "tranquil" has been the most frequent type of intervention used with adult surgical patients. Music interventions for children have been more varied and include live interactive music, musical preoperative teaching, and relaxation techniques paired with music, in both individual and group sessions. This chapter discusses research and current practices using music as a pediatric surgical intervention and includes clinical recommendations for pediatric music therapists.

RATIONALE FOR PREOPERATIVE INTERVENTIONS WITH PEDIATRIC PATIENTS

Why do children need preoperative interventions? Very simply, they get scared. Often they do not know or understand what is going on, why they have to be at the hospital, and why they have to wear a gown that does not even cover them up. They wonder who all the people wearing masks are and why they are poking around with needles and tubes. Some children have already had one or more surgical experiences and may question if the outcome will be the same as the last. Will it hurt? How long will it be before full recovery? Will there be a full recovery? Children's thoughts and emotions can sometimes be overlooked or minimized when serious procedures need to occur.

Anxiety during the preoperative period generally arises from factors such as fear, unfamiliarity and unpredictability of the hospital environment, and pre-existing stressors. Children are often afraid of pain, medications and needles, separation from their parents, disfigurement, loss of control over their body and environment, death, and the unknown (Bossert, 1994; Melamed, Meyer, Gee, & Soule, 1993; O'Dougherty & Brown, 1990; Pinto & Hollandsworth, 1989). Past negative experiences with surgery also play a significant role in the amount of discomfort and anticipatory anxiety a child may feel.

Most pediatric patients experience uncertainty regarding the hospital environment, especially during their first admission. Medical facilities and pediatric hospitals often establish "kid-friendly" rooms with wall murals, toys, cartoons, games, and stuffed animals. This type of environment can certainly aid in reducing anxiety associated with the hospital itself, but children still know they are in an unfamiliar place. Some children will require additional support services that help diminish the unfamiliarity and unpredictability experienced by children during a hospital admission or outpatient surgical experience.

Outside stressors that may occur prior to hospital admission, such as familial issues, difficulties at school, or challenges with friends also contribute to preoperative anxiety. Parents and family members often have as much, if not more, stress about the surgical experience and its outcome. Emotions are contagious, and parental anxiety has been found to effect a child's anxiety level—a phenomenon referred to as emotional contagion (Melnyk, 1995; Siegel & Hudson, 1992; Whelan & Kirby, 2000). Interventions that address parental anxiety have a direct impact on the amount of anxiety experienced by the pediatric patient.

Children may have to miss school and can easily fall behind in academics. In addition to academic concerns, anxiety can lead to periods of developmental regression where the child may revert to behaviors associated with an earlier stage of development (Bossert, 1994; Siegel & Hudson, 1992). This is viewed as a normal coping response; however, prolonged periods of regressive behavior are cause for concern and warrant intervention. In isolation each of these factors can be anxiety-producing, but patients and families are often faced with multiple sources of stress which further accentuate the level of preoperative anxiety experienced by pediatric patients and their families.

If preoperative anxiety is not addressed and reduced, manifestations such as combative behavior can occur. Combative behavior can be displayed in the form of hitting, kicking, pulling away from staff, taking out IVs, refusing to cooperate, crying, and screaming, which can result in the need for more preoperative sedation or anesthesia (Lumley, Melamed, & Abeles, 1993; Whelan & Kirby, 1998). The more sedation that is used, the longer it takes for the patient to wake up in recovery, and the more side effects the child is likely to experience. Another potential result of not addressing preoperative anxiety is establishing or perpetuating a cycle of fear for pediatric patients who have multiple surgeries in their future.

Other factors associated with hospitalization warrant a need for preoperative interventions as well. Patient and parental perceptions of the surgical experience are very important to hospital administration and staff. Each procedure leading up to the surgery itself can compound the trauma of hospitalization for a child and family. Children rarely have a choice in the matter of when and where surgical procedures take place. A child's loss of control over his/her body or environment contributes to the trauma. Preoperative interventions for pediatric patients are designed to reduce anxiety and fear, normalize the environment, increase sense of control, improve perception of procedures, and increase relaxation.

Music interventions have been found to be an effective and noninvasive method for managing anxiety and behavioral distress associated with the surgical experience. Standley's (1986) meta-analysis reported that 54 out of 55 measured variables were improved by music interventions in the medical setting. Variables measured included physiological and psychological responses to music such as reduction in perioperative stress hormones, decreased anxiety, and increased sleep.

PREOPERATIVE MUSIC THERAPY INTERVENTIONS

While research with adults has primarily utilized music as passive listening, nearly all of the pediatric literature reflects a more interactive approach. These interventions fall into three basic categories: active interventions, preoperative education, and relaxation techniques.

Active Interventions

What do active music therapy interventions look like? In order to reduce anxiety associated with the unfamiliar and unpredictable characteristics of the hospital, music therapists use music that children find both familiar and enjoyable. A variety of melodic and percussive instruments and interactive visual aids are used to actively engage children in nonthreatening, developmentally appropriate activities. By engaging children actively, the music therapist is able to redirect the child's attention away from anxiety producing stimuli in the environment. Guitars, keyboards, tambourines, drums, omnichords, shakers, maracas, and bells are some of the instruments utilized during interactive sessions. Interactive visual aids often include puppets, stuffed animals, books, toys, videos, costumes, and masks. Active music interventions are selected and designed to match the behavioral needs of the pediatric patient. If the child is withdrawn or exhibiting signs of behavioral distress, the music and interactive qualities of the music will begin at a slower tempo, gradually moving the child toward a more interactive state. If the child is more active, interventions may seek to diminish the child's activity level or maintain their focus of attention in a central activity. This is generally accomplished by matching the child's activity level through attributes of the music, as well as the interactive qualities of the selected activity. These interventions function to reduce anxiety by engaging the child in a meaningful activity that is fun, safe, and familiar.

Two studies investigating the use of interactive, live music interventions to diminish preoperative anxiety in pediatric patients support the use of music. Aldridge (1993) used live music therapy activities designed to reduce anxiety and promote self-expression, security, and familiarity with pediatric surgical patients. Results from the study indicated that parent-rated levels of patients' anxiety decreased, and comfort levels increased (Aldridge, 1993). Another study using 20 minutes of live, interactive music therapy with children 3–10 years old yielded significant decreases in preoperative anxiety for pediatric surgical patients in the music group (Scheve, 2002).

Preoperative Education

There is a large body of research literature that has established the importance of preoperative teaching (Lynch, 1994; Melamed et al., 1993; Pinto & Hollandsworth, 1989; Twardosz, Weddle, Borden, & Stevens, 1986; Whelan & Kirby, 1998, 2000). With children, preoperative teaching has been most successful when an interactive, hands-on approach is adopted. This often includes touring the operating room, as well as having the opportunity to view and manipulate materials that will be used on the day of surgery (i.e., anesthesia mask, gowns, shoe covers, or syringes).

Chetta (1981) investigated an intervention that combined music with preoperative information to reduce anxiety in children. Chetta studied the effects of two music interventions on preoperative anxiety in children ages 3–8; preoperative education combined with live music (using songs to reinforce the information), and musical preoperative education plus music therapy the morning of surgery. All sessions were 20–30 minutes in length and included allowing the children to give a doll a shot. The music group that received live music therapy the morning of surgery experienced significant reductions in anxiety and were rated as more relaxed during preoperative injections when compared with participants in the control and musical preoperative education groups.

Relaxation Techniques

While younger children use behavioral strategies to cope with anxiety, older children and adolescents are cognitively capable of using more passive approaches for anxiety reduction, such as various relaxation techniques. Music assisted relaxation has been employed to reduce preoperative anxiety in surgical patients 8–20 years old (Robb, Nichols, Rutan, Bishop, & Parker, 1995). The music interventions occurred the night before surgery and 1 hour prior to surgery, and consisted of 30–50 minutes of deep diaphragmatic breathing, progressive muscle relaxation, and patient-generated imagery, all paired with music. Results indicated that while there was no significant change in physiologic measures, state anxiety was significantly decreased in the music group. In this study, the relaxation techniques used during the preoperative period were continued as the patient was transferred from their room into the surgical suite. These interventions were used to support patients during anesthesia induction; however, data were not collected during the perioperative period.

RATIONALE FOR POSTOPERATIVE INTERVENTIONS

The postoperative period generally includes two stages: emergence from anesthesia in the PACU or PICU, and time spent on the pediatric floor awaiting discharge. Postoperative concerns do not tremendously differ from preoperative concerns for pediatric patients. Anxiety and discomfort related to the environment and fear of the unknown are still present, but the postoperative period introduces pain and confusion not necessarily experienced prior to surgery. Anesthesia, sedatives, and pain medications often have adverse side effects for pediatric patients such as dizziness, nightmares, headaches, insomnia, respiratory depression, cardiovascular distress, confusion, hallucinations, nausea and vomiting, personality changes, and acute psychosis (Sifton, 2000).

During the latter stage of the postoperative period, patients begin to experience acceptance or denial of the surgical outcome(s), frustration during the rehabilitation process, and anxiety regarding extended hospitalization and the future. Children often have to be integrated back into school and social activities, having been absent due to surgery and hospitalization. Family dynamics may have changed as well. Music therapy interventions can target these obstacles and improve the postoperative period for pediatric patients.

POSTOPERATIVE MUSIC THERAPY INTERVENTIONS

Postoperative music interventions with pediatric patients generally focus on pain reduction. The same type of interventions employed with preoperative patients can be used postoperatively. Siegel (1983) examined the use of music-based relaxation strategies during the postoperative period. Specifically, the author measured the effectiveness of recorded music paired with progressive muscle relaxation and guided imagery on frequency of pain medication requests, vital signs, and pain reports by patients and nurses. The music group requested pain medication significantly less frequently than the control group (Siegel, 1983). As an active intervention, Bradt (2001) utilized music entrainment and the iso-principle to match the patients' pain level with live music to reduce postoperative pain in patients 8–19 years old. Results from the study indicated significant outcomes for decreased pain, mood elevation, and perceived levels of control for postoperative music therapy sessions (Bradt, 2001). Multiple studies examining the use of music-based interventions to reduce postoperative anxiety have been conducted with adults (Crago, 1980; Good et al., 2001; Mullooly, Levin, & Feldman, 1988). This body of research provides a foundation for future studies that directly examine the efficacy of these interventions for pediatric populations. Additional goals for postoperative pediatric patients are mentioned in the clinical recommendations section at the end of this chapter.

MUSIC THERAPY WITH PARENTS AND FAMILIES

Few researchers have studied the effect of music therapy on parents and families of pediatric surgical patients. Oggenfuss (2001) used live interactive music therapy for children awaiting surgery and measured the parents' preoperative anxiety levels. Music therapy sessions occurred approximately 30 minutes prior to surgery, and parents were then asked to rate both their anxiety levels and their perceptions of their child's anxiety. Although the results were not statistically significant, a trend suggested that parents' anxiety was reduced and 100% of parents surveyed stated that the music therapy was beneficial for their child (Oggenfuss, 2001).

The effectiveness of live music on anxiety levels of persons waiting in a surgical waiting room yielded significant results (Jarred, 2003). Relaxation levels were significantly increased for subjects who listened to music they requested. Subjects who were able to choose the specific songs they heard reported significantly more enjoyment of the music than the group that listened to music without choosing specific songs. All 121 participants in the two music groups reported that live music therapy in the surgical waiting room is a service they think the hospital should offer (Jarred, 2003).

CONCLUDING REMARKS

The use of music therapy interventions with pediatric surgical patients is an effective way to significantly improve the surgical and hospital experience for both patients and families. Research supports the use of active interventions, surgical education, and relaxation techniques to reduce anxiety and possibly the amount of sedation and pain medication required by the patient. This body of research has also documented the benefits of music interventions to increase relaxation and improve perception of hospitalization during the pre- and postoperative periods. Currently, there is a limited amount of empirical research that has been conducted during the perioperative period with pediatric patients. Emerging studies conducted with neonates and adults in this area forecast that music therapy may be effective in reducing anxiety and the amount of medications required during surgery (Joyce, Keck, & Gerkensmeyer, 2001; Marchette, Main, Redick, Bagg, & Leatherland, 1991; Oyama, Sato, Kudo, Spintge, & Droh, 1983; Tanioka et al., 1985). The reader is referred to a list of clinical recommendations provided at the end of this chapter. The clinical recommendations list includes suggested music therapy goals and objectives for the pre-, peri-, and postoperative periods. Future research in music assisted surgery requires joint efforts between music therapists and medical staff to establish music therapy as standard care for pediatric surgical patients.

CLINICAL RECOMMENDATIONS

Preoperative Goals

- decrease anxiety and separation fear
- increase relaxation
- increase perception of control
- decrease perception of pain
- normalize the environment
- increase family interaction
- decrease the trauma of hospitalization
- increase perception of procedure and hospitalization
- increase quality of life

Preoperative Objectives

- use live music whenever possible
- "surgery buddies": interactive and stimulating music therapy
- isoprinciple: turn shy and scared kids into interactive and animated kids
- patient preferred music: let the patient choose songs and activities for more effective sessions and to give the patient control
- preoperative education: involve music and role playing for preparation
- relaxation techniques: progressive muscle and guided imagery paired with music
- psychological preparation: counseling and separation coping

Perioperative Goals

- decrease anxiety and separation fear
- increase relaxation
- decrease pain and physiological distress
- increase perception of procedure
- decrease amount of sedation required
- increase coping and relaxation for family

Perioperative Objectives

- use live music if possible
- pre- to perioperative transition: be with the patient as long as the medical staff will allow to give the patient support during separation from parents and family
- headphones: familiar music with therapeutic suggestions, guided imagery
- music therapy in the waiting room for parents and families
- use preferred music: encourage the family to choose songs they like in order to be effective in distraction/relaxation and to give them control

Postoperative Goals

- decrease anxiety
- decrease pain and physiological distress
- increase relaxation, decreasing amount of pain medication required
- decrease nausea
- normalize the environment
- increase family interaction
- decrease trauma of hospitalization
- increase perception of procedure and hospitalization
- increase motivation and endurance during rehabilitation
- decrease length of stay
- increase quality of life

Postoperative Objectives

- use live music whenever possible
- PACU, PICU, pediatric floor: interactive and stimulating music therapy
- iso-principle: decrease pain and increase relaxation
- patient preferred music: let the patient choose songs and activities for more effective sessions and to give the patient control
- postoperative education: plan and prepare for future surgeries if applicable, pain management
- physical therapy: structure music to increase motivation and compliance
- relaxation techniques: progressive muscle and guided imagery paired with music
- coping and counseling: dealing with physiological and psychological changes resulting from surgery, and goal setting
- attend interdisciplinary team meetings/rounds: always be informed about your patients and report progress or concerns

REFERENCES

Aldridge, K. (1993). The use of music to relieve pre-operational anxiety in children attending day surgery. *The Australian Journal of Music Therapy, 4*, 19–35.

Allen, K., Golden, L. H., Izzo, J. L., Jr., Ching, M. I., Forrest, A., Niles, C. R., Niswander, P. R., & Barlow, J. C. (2001). Normalization of hypertensive responses during ambulatory surgical stress by perioperative music. *Psychosomatic Medicine, 63*(3), 487–492.

Bossert, E. (1994). Factors influencing the coping of hospitalized school-age children. *Journal of Pediatric Nursing, 9*, 299–306.

Bradt, J. (2001). *The effects of music entrainment on postoperative pain perception in pediatric patients*. Unpublished doctoral dissertation, Temple University, Philadelphia.

Byers, J. F., & Smyth, K. A. (1997). Effect of a music intervention on noise annoyance, heart rate, and blood pressure in cardiac surgery patients. *American Journal of Critical Care, 6* (3),

183–191.

Chetta, H. D. (1981). The effect of music and desensitization on preoperative anxiety in children. *Journal of Music Therapy, 18*(2), 74–87.

Crago, B. (1980). *Reducing the stress of hospitalization for open heart surgery*. Unpublished doctoral dissertation, University of Massachussetts, Amherst.

Good, M., Stanton-Hicks, M., Grass, J. A., Anderson, G. C, Lai, H., Roykulcharoen, V., & Adler, P. A. (2001). Relaxation and music reduce postsurgical pain. *Journal of Advanced Nursing, 33*(2), 208–215.

Jarred, J. D. (2003). *The effect of live music on anxiety levels of persons waiting in a surgical waiting room as measured by self-report*. Unpublished master's thesis, The Florida State University, Tallahassee.

Joyce, B. A., Keck, J. F., & Gerkensmeyer, J. (2001). Evaluation of pain management interventions for neonatal circumcision pain. *Journal of Pediatric Health Care, 15*(3), 105–114.

Kaempf, G., & Amodei, G. (1989). The effect of music on anxiety. *AORN Journal, 50*(1), 112–118.

Lepage, C., Drolet, P., Girard, M., Grenier, Y., & DeGayne, R. (2001). Music decreases sedative requirements during spinal anesthesia. *Anesthesia & Analgesia, 93*(4), 912–916.

Locsin, R. (1981). The effect of music on the pain of selected post-operative patients. *Journal of Advanced Nursing, 6*, 19–25.

Lumley, M. A., Melamed, B. G., & Abeles, L. A. (1993). Predicting children's presurgical anxiety and subsequent behavior changes. *Journal of Pediatric Psychology, 18*(4), 481–497.

Lynch, M. (1994). Preparing children for day surgery. *Children's Health Care, 23*(2), 75–85.

Marchette, L., Main, R., Redick, E., Bagg, A., & Leatherland, J. (1991). Pain reduction interventions during neonatal circumcision. *Nursing Research, 40*(4), 241–244.

Melamed, B. G., Meyer, R., Gee, C., & Soule, L. (1993). The influence of time and type of preparation on children's adjustment to hospitalization. In M. C. Roberts & G. P. Koocher (Eds.), *Readings in pediatric psychology* (pp. 223–236). New York: Plenum Press.

Melnyk, B. M. (1995). Parental coping with childhood hospitalization: A theoretical framework to guide research and clinical interventions. *Maternal-Child Nursing Journal, 23*(4), 123–131.

Mullooly, V. M., Levin, R. F., & Feldman, H. R. (1988). Music for postoperative pain and anxiety. *The Journal of the New York State Nurses Association, 19*(2), 4–7.

Nilsson, U., Rawal, N., Enqvist, B., & Unosson, M. (2003). Analgesia following music and therapeutic suggestions in the PACU in ambulatory surgery; a randomized controlled trial. *Acta Anaesthesia Scandinavica, 47*(3), 278–283.

O'Dougherty, M., & Brown, R. T. (1990). The stress of childhood illness. In A. L. Eugene (Ed.), *Childhood stress* (pp. 326–349). New York: Wiley.

Oggenfuss (2001). *Pediatric surgery patients and parent anxiety: Can live music therapy effectively reduce stress and anxiety levels while waiting to go to surgery?* Unpublished master's thesis, The Florida State University, Tallahassee.

Oyama, T., Sato, Y., Kudo, M., Spintge, R., & Droh, R. (1983). Effect of anxiolytic music on endocrine function in surgical patients. In R. Droh & R. Spintge (Eds.), *Angst, schmerz, musik in der anasthesie* (pp. 147–152). Basel, Germany: Editiones Roche.

Pinto, R. P., & Hollandsworth, J. G. (1989). Using videotape modeling to prepare children psychologically for surgery: Influence of parents and costs versus benefits of providing preparation services. *Health Psychology, 8*(1), 79–95.

Robb, S. L., Nichols, R. J., Rutan, R. L., Bishop, B. L., & Parker, J. C. (1995). The effects of music assisted relaxation on preoperative anxiety. *Journal of Music Therapy, 32*(1), 2–21.

Sanderson, S. (1986). *The effect of music on reducing preoperative anxiety and postoperative anxiety and pain in the recovery room*. Unpublished master's thesis, The Florida State University, Tallahassee.

Scheve, A. (2002). *The effect of music therapy intervention on pre-operative anxiety of pediatric patients as measured by self report.* Unpublished master's thesis, The Florida State University, Tallahassee.

Siegel, S. L. (1983). *The use of music as treatment in pain perception with post-surgical patients in a pediatric hospital.* Unpublished master's thesis, University of Miami, Coral Gables, Florida.

Siegel, L. J., & Hudson, B. O. (1992). Hospitalization and medical care of children. In C. E. Walker & M. C. Roberts (Eds.), *Handbook of clinical child psychology* (2nd ed., pp. 845–858). New York: John Wiley & Sons.

Sifton, D. W. (2000). *The PDR pocket guide to prescription drugs* (4th ed.). New York: Pocket Books.

Standley, J. (1986). Music research in medical/dental treatment: A meta-analysis and clinical applications. *Journal of Music Therapy, 23*(2), 56–122.

Standley, J. (2000). Music research in medical treatment. In *Effectiveness of music therapy procedures: Documentation of research and clinical practice* (3rd ed., pp. 1–64). Silver Spring, MD: American Music Therapy Association.

Tanioka, F., Takazawa, T., Kamata, S., Kudo, M., Matsuki, A., & Oyama, T. (1985). Hormonal effect of anxiolytic music in patients during surgical operations under epidural anaesthesia. In R. Droh & R. Spintge (Eds.), *Angst, schmerz, musik in der anasthesie* (pp. 147–152). Basel, Germany: Editiones Roche.

Taylor, D. (1981). Music in general hospital treatment from 1900 to 1950. *Journal of Music Therapy, 18*, 62–73.

Twardosz, S., Weddle, K., Borden, L., & Stevens, E. (1986). A comparison of three methods of preparing children for surgery. *Behavior Therapy, 17*(1), 14–25.

Updike, P. A., & Charles, D. M. (1987). Music Rx: Physiological and emotional responses to taped music programs of preoperative patients awaiting plastic surgery. *Annals of Plastic Surgery, 19*(1), 29–33.

Walters, C. L. (1996). The psychological and physiological effects of vibrotactile stimulation, via a Somatron, on patients awaiting scheduled gynecological surgery. *Journal of Music Therapy, 33*(4), 261–287.

Whelan, T. A., & Kirby, R. J. (1998). Advantages for children and their families of psychological preparation for hospitalization and surgery. *Journal of Family Studies, 4*(1), 35–51.

Whelan, T. A., & Kirby, R. J. (2000). Parent adjustment to a child's hospitalization. *Journal of Family Studies, 6*(1), 46–64.

RELATED LITERATURE

Effect of Music on Physiological Responses

Allen, K., Golden, L.H., Izzo, J. L., Jr., Ching, M. I., Forrest, A., Niles, C. R., Niswander, P. R., & Barlow, J. C. (2001). Normalization of hypertensive responses during ambulatory surgical stress by perioperative music. *Psychosomatic Medicine, 63*(3), 487–492.

Augustin, P., & Harris, A. A. (1996). Effect of music on ambulatory surgery patients' preoperative anxiety. *AORN Journal, 63*(4), 750–758.

Barnason, S., Zimmerman, L., & Nieveen, J. (1995). The effects of music interventions on anxiety in the patient after coronary artery bypass grafting. *Heart & Lung, 24*(2), 124–132.

Blankfield, R. P., Zyzanski, S. J., Flocke, S. A., Alemango, S., & Scheurman, K. (1995). Taped therapeutic suggestions and taped music as adjuncts in the care of coronary-artery-bypass patients. *American Journal of Clinical Hypnosis, 37*(3), 32–42.

Byers, J. F., & Smyth, K. A. (1997). Effect of a music intervention on noise annoyance, heart rate, and blood pressure in cardiac surgery patients. *American Journal of Critical Care, 6*(3), 183–191.

Heitz, L., Symreng, T., & Scamman, F. (1992). Effect of music therapy in the postanesthesia care unit: A nursing intervention. *Journal of Post Anesthesia Nursing, 7*(1), 22–31.

Kaempf, G., & Amodei, G. (1989). The effect of music on anxiety. *AORN Journal, 50*(1), 112–118.

Locsin, R. (1981). The effect of music on the pain of selected post-operative patients. *Journal of Advanced Nursing, 6*, 19–25.

Miluk-Kolasa, B., Obminski, Z., Stupnicki, R., & Golec, L. (1994). Effects of music treatment on salivary cortisol in patients exposed to pre-surgical stress. *Experimental and Clinical Endocrinology, 102*, 118–120.

Oyama, T., Sato, Y., Kudo, M., Spintge, R., & Droh, R. (1983). Effect of anxiolytic music on endocrine function in surgical patients. In R. Droh & R. Spintge (Eds.), *Angst, schmerz, musik in der anasthesie* (pp. 147–152). Basel, Germany: Editiones Roche.

Sanderson, S. (1986). *The effect of music on reducing preoperative anxiety and postoperative anxiety and pain in the recovery room*. Unpublished master's thesis, The Florida State University, Tallahassee.

Steelman, V. M. (1990). Intraoperative music therapy. *AORN Journal, 52*(5), 1026–1034.

Tanioka, F., Takazawa, T., Kamata, S., Kudo, M., Matsuki, A., & Oyama, T. (1985). Hormonal effect of anxiolytic music in patients during surgical operations under epidural anaesthesia. In R. Droh & R. Spintge (Eds.), *Angst, schmerz, musik in der anasthesie* (pp. 147–152). Basel, Germany: Editiones Roche.

Updike, P. A., & Charles, D. M. (1987). Music Rx: Physiological and emotional responses to taped music programs of preoperative patients awaiting plastic surgery. *Annals of Plastic Surgery, 19*(1), 29–33.

Walters, C. L. (1996). The psychological and physiological effects of vibrotactile stimulation, via a Somatron, on patients awaiting scheduled gynecological surgery. *Journal of Music Therapy, 33*(4), 261–287.

Whisnant, R. (2003). Soothing sounds—Music therapy can be used during surgery to reduce pain, anxiety, and even the level of anesthesia needed. *Minnesota Medicine, 86*(2), 38–40.

Zimmerman, L., Nieveen, J., Barnason, S., & Schmaderer, M. (1996). The effects of music interventions on postoperative pain and sleep in coronary artery bypass graft (CABG) patients. *Scholarly Inquiry for Nursing Practice: An International Journal, 10*(2), 153–174.

Effect of Music on Psychological Responses

Allen, K., Golden, L. H., Izzo, J. L., Jr., Ching, M. I., Forrest, A., Niles, C. R., Niswander, P. R., & Barlow, J. C. (2001). Normalization of hypertensive responses during ambulatory surgical stress by perioperative music. *Psychosomatic Medicine, 63*(3), 487–492.

Barnason, S., Zimmerman, L., & Nieveen, J. (1995). The effects of music interventions on anxiety in the patient after coronary artery bypass grafting. *Heart & Lung, 24*(2), 124–132.

Blankfield, R. P., Zyzanski, S. J., Flocke, S. A., Alemango, S., & Scheurman, K. (1995). Taped therapeutic suggestions and taped music as adjuncts in the care of coronary-artery-bypass patients. *American Journal of Clinical Hypnosis, 37*(3), 32–42.

Byers, J. F., & Smyth, K. A. (1997). Effect of a music intervention on noise annoyance, heart rate, and blood pressure in cardiac surgery patients. *American Journal of Critical Care, 6*(3), 183–191.

Cowan, D. S. (1991). Music therapy in the surgical arena. *Music Therapy Perspectives, 9*, 42–45.

Crago, B. (1980). *Reducing the stress of hospitalization for open heart surgery*. Unpublished doctoral dissertation, University of Massachussetts, Amherst.

Gaberson, K. B. (1995). The effect of humorous and musical distraction on preoperative anxiety. *AORN Journal, 62*(5), 784–791.

Good, M. (1995). A comparison of the effects of jaw relaxation and music on postoperative pain. *Nursing Research, 44*(1), 52–57.

Good, M., Stanton-Hicks, M., Grass, J. A., Anderson, G. C, Lai, H., Roykulcharoen, V., & Adler, P. A. (2001). Relaxation and music reduce postsurgical pain. *Journal of Advanced Nursing, 33*(2), 208–215.

Goroszeniuk, T., & Morgan, B. (1984). Music during epidural caesarean section. *The Practitioner, 228*, 441–443.

Heitz, L., Symreng, T., & Scamman, F. (1992). Effect of music therapy in the postanesthesia care unit: A nursing intervention. *Journal of Post Anesthesia Nursing, 7*(1), 22–31.

Kaempf, G., & Amodei, G. (1989). The effect of music on anxiety. *AORN Journal, 50*(1), 112–118.

Kumar, A., Bajaj, A., Sarkar, P., & Grover, V. K. (1992). The effect of music on ketamine induces emergence phenomena. *Anaesthesia, 47*, 438–439.

Light, G., Love, D., Benson, D., & Morch, E. (1954). Music in surgery. *Current Researchers in Anesthesia and Analgesia, 33*, 258–264.

Locsin, R. (1981). The effect of music on the pain of selected post-operative patients. *Journal of Advanced Nursing, 6*, 19–25.

MacClelland, D.C. (1979). Music in the operating room. *AORN Journal, 29*(2), 252–260.

Miluk-Kolasa, B., Klodecka-Rozalska, J., & Stupnicki, R. (2002). The effect of music listening on perioperative anxiety levels in adult surgical patients. *Polish Psychological Bulletin, 33*(2), 55–60.

Miluk-Kolasa, B., Obminski, Z., Stupnicki, R., & Golec, L. (1994). Effects of music treatment on salivary cortisol in patients exposed to pre-surgical stress. *Experimental and Clinical Endocrinology, 102*, 118–120.

Moss, V. (1988). Music and the surgical patient. *AORN Journal, 48*, 64–69.

Mullooly, V. M., Levin, R. F., & Feldman, H. R. (1988). Music for postoperative pain and anxiety. *The Journal of the New York State Nurses Association, 19*(2), 4–7.

Nilsson, U., Rawal, N., Enqvist, B., & Unosson, M. (2003). Analgesia following music and therapeutic suggestions in the PACU in ambulatory surgery; a randomized controlled trial. *Acta Anaesthesia Scandinavica, 47*(3), 278–283.

Oyama, T., Sato, Y., Kudo, M., Spintge, R., & Droh, R. (1983). Effect of anxiolytic music on endocrine function in surgical patients. In R. Droh & R. Spintge (Eds.), *Angst, schmerz, musik in der anasthesie* (pp. 147–152). Basel, Germany: Editiones Roche.

Sanderson, S. (1986). *The effect of music on reducing preoperative anxiety and postoperative anxiety and pain in the recovery room*. Unpublished master's thesis, The Florida State University, Tallahassee.

Stevens, K. (1990). Patients' perceptions of music during surgery. *Journal of Advanced Nursing, 15*, 1045–1051.

Tanioka, F., Takazawa, T., Kamata, S., Kudo, M., Matsuki, A., & Oyama, T. (1985). Hormonal effect of anxiolytic music in patients during surgical operations under epidural anaesthesia. In R. Droh & R. Spintge (Eds.), *Angst, schmerz, musik in der anasthesie* (pp. 147–152). Basel, Germany: Editiones Roche.

Toupin, L., & Ames, B. B. (2002). Snorkel makes surgery calmer for kids: Anesthesia mask mixes music, video games, and choice of colors. *Design News, 57*(18), 62–65.

Taylor, L. K., Kuttler, K. L., Parks, T. A., & Milton, D. (1998). The effect of music in the postanesthesia care unit on pain levels in women who have had abdominal hysterectomies. *Journal of PeriAnesthesia Nursing, 13*(2), 88–94.

Updike, P. A., & Charles, D. M. (1987). Music Rx: Physiological and emotional responses to taped music programs of preoperative patients awaiting plastic surgery. *Annals of Plastic Surgery, 19*(1), 29–33.

Walters, C. L. (1996). The psychological and physiological effects of vibrotactile stimulation, via a Somatron, on patients awaiting scheduled gynecological surgery. *Journal of Music Therapy, 33*(4), 261–287.

Zimmerman, L., Nieveen, J., Barnason, S., & Schmaderer, M. (1996). The effects of music interventions on postoperative pain and slep in coronary artery bypass graft (CABG) patients. *Scholarly Inquiry for Nursing Practice: An International Journal, 10*(2), 153–174.

Effect of Music on Preoperative Anxiety

Gaberson, K. B. (1995). The effect of humorous and musical distraction on preoperative anxiety. *AORN Journal, 62*(5), 784–791.

Kaempf, G., & Amodei, G. (1989). The effect of music on anxiety. *AORN Journal, 50*(1), 112–118.

Miluk-Kolasa, B., Obminski, Z., Stupnicki, R., & Golec, L. (1994). Effects of music treatment on salivary cortisol in patients exposed to pre-surgical stress. *Experimental and Clinical*

Endocrinology, 102, 118–120.

Sanderson, S. (1986). *The effect of music on reducing preoperative anxiety and postoperative anxiety and pain in the recovery room*. Unpublished master's thesis, The Florida State University, Tallahassee.

Toupin, L., & Ames, B. B. (2002). Snorkel makes surgery calmer for kids: anesthesia mask mixes music, video games, and choice of colors. *Design News, 57*(18), 62–65.

Walters, C. L. (1996). The psychological and physiological effects of vibrotactile stimulation, via a Somatron, on patients awaiting scheduled gynecological surgery. *Journal of Music Therapy, 33*(4), 261–287.

Effect of Music on the Amount of Anesthesia or Pain Medications Required Peri- or Postoperatively

Crago, B. (1980). *Reducing the stress of hospitalization for open heart surgery*. Unpublished doctoral dissertation, University of Massachusetts, Amherst.

Good, M. (1995). A comparison of the effects of jaw relaxation and music on postoperative pain. *Nursing Research, 44*(1), 52–57.

Heitz, L., Symreng, T., & Scamman, F. (1992). Effect of music therapy in the postanesthesia care unit: A nursing intervention. *Journal of Post Anesthesia Nursing, 7*(1), 22–31.

Lepage, C., Drolet, P., Girard, M., Grenier, Y., & DeGayne, R. (2001). Music decreases sedative requirements during spinal anesthesia. *Anesthesia & Analgesia, 93*(4), 912–916.

Locsin, R. (1981). The effect of music on the pain of selected post-operative patients. *Journal of Advanced Nursing, 6*, 19–25.

Nilsson, U., Rawal, N., Enqvist, B., & Unosson, M. (2003). Analgesia following music and therapeutic suggestions in the PACU in ambulatory surgery; a randomized controlled trial. *Acta Anaesthesia Scandinavica, 47*(3), 278–283.

Sanderson, S. (1986). *The effect of music on reducing preoperative anxiety and postoperative anxiety and pain in the recovery room*. Unpublished master's thesis, The Florida State University, Tallahassee.

Whisnant, R. (2003). Soothing sounds—Music therapy can be used during surgery to reduce pain, anxiety, and even the level of anesthesia needed. *Minnesota Medicine, 86*(2), 38–40.

Use of Preoperative Music

Allen, K., Golden, L. H., Izzo, J. L., Jr., Ching, M. I., Forrest, A., Niles, C. R., Niswander, P. R., & Barlow, J. C. (2001). Normalization of hypertensive responses during ambulatory surgical stress by perioperative music. *Psychosomatic Medicine, 63*(3), 487–492.

Augustin, P., & Harris, A. A. (1996). Effect of music on ambulatory surgery patients' preoperative anxiety. *AORN Journal, 63*(4), 750–758.

Gaberson, K. B. (1995). The effect of humorous and musical distraction on preoperative anxiety. *AORN Journal, 62*(5), 784–791.

Kaempf, G., & Amodei, G. (1989). The effect of music on anxiety. *AORN Journal, 50*(1), 112–118.

Miluk-Kolasa, B., Obminski, Z., Stupnicki, R., & Golec, L. (1994). Effects of music treatment on salivary cortisol in patients exposed to pre-surgical stress. *Experimental and Clinical*

Endocrinology, 102, 118–120.

Sanderson, S. (1986). *The effect of music on reducing preoperative anxiety and postoperative anxiety and pain in the recovery room*. Unpublished master's thesis, The Florida State University, Tallahassee.

Toupin, L., & Ames, B. B. (2002). Snorkel makes surgery calmer for kids: anesthesia mask mixes music, video games, and choice of colors. *Design News, 57*(18), 62–65.

Updike, P. A., & Charles, D. M. (1987). Music Rx: Physiological and emotional responses to taped music programs of preoperative patients awaiting plastic surgery. *Annals of Plastic Surgery, 19*(1), 29–33.

Walters, C. L. (1996). The psychological and physiological effects of vibrotactile stimulation, via a Somatron, on patients awaiting scheduled gynecological surgery. *Journal of Music Therapy, 33*(4), 261–287.

Use of Perioperative Music

Allen, K., Golden, L. H., Izzo, J. L., Jr., Ching, M. I., Forrest, A., Niles, C. R., Niswander, P. R., & Barlow, J. C. (2001). Normalization of hypertensive responses during ambulatory surgical stress by perioperative music. *Psychosomatic Medicine, 63*(3), 487–492.

Blankfield, R. P., Zyzanski, S. J., Flocke, S. A., Alemango, S., & Scheurman, K. (1995). Taped therapeutic suggestions and taped music as adjuncts in the care of coronary-artery-bypass patients. *American Journal of Clinical Hypnosis, 37*(3), 32–42.

Cowan, D. S. (1991). Music therapy in the surgical arena. *Music Therapy Perspectives, 9*, 42–45.

Goroszeniuk, T., & Morgan, B. (1984). Music during epidural caesarean section. *The Practitioner, 228*, 441–443.

Kumar, A., Bajaj, A., Sarkar, P., & Grover, V. K. (1992). The effect of music on ketamine induces emergence phenomena. *Anaesthesia, 47*, 438–439.

Lepage, C., Drolet, P., Girard, M., Grenier, Y., & DeGayne, R. (2001). Music decreases sedative requirements during spinal anesthesia. *Anesthesia & Analgesia, 93*(4), 912–916.

Light, G., Love, D., Benson, D., & Morch, E. (1954). Music in surgery. *Current Researchers in Anesthesia and Analgesia, 33*, 258–264.

MacClelland, D. C. (1979). Music in the operating room. *AORN Journal, 29*(2), 252–260.

Miluk-Kolasa, B., Klodecka-Rozalska, J., & Stupnicki, R. (2002). The effect of music listening on perioperative anxiety levels in adult surgical patients. *Polish Psychological Bulletin, 33*(2), 55–60.

Moss, V. (1988). Music and the surgical patient. *AORN Journal, 48*, 64–69.

Oyama, T., Sato, Y., Kudo, M., Spintge, R., & Droh, R. (1983). Effect of anxiolytic music on endocrine function in surgical patients. In R. Droh & R. Spintge (Eds.), *Angst, schmerz, musik in der anasthesie* (pp. 147–152). Basel, Germany: Editiones Roche.

Steelman, V. M. (1990). Intraoperative music therapy. *AORN Journal, 52*(5), 1026–1034.

Stevens, K. (1990). Patients' perceptions of music during surgery. *Journal of Advanced Nursing, 15*, 1045–1051.

Tanioka, F., Takazawa, T., Kamata, S., Kudo, M., Matsuki, A., & Oyama, T. (1985). Hormonal effect of anxiolytic music in patients during surgical operations under epidural anaesthesia. In R. Droh & R. Spintge (Eds.), *Angst, schmerz, musik in der anasthesie* (pp. 147–152). Basel,

Germany: Editiones Roche.

Whisnant, R. (2003). Soothing sounds—Music therapy can be used during surgery to reduce pain, anxiety, and even the level of anesthesia needed. *Minnesota Medicine, 86*(2), 38–40.

Use of Postoperative Music

Allen, K., Golden, L. H., Izzo, J. L., Jr., Ching, M. I., Forrest, A., Niles, C. R., Niswander, P. R., & Barlow, J. C. (2001). Normalization of hypertensive responses during ambulatory surgical stress by perioperative music. *Psychosomatic Medicine, 63*(3), 487–492.

Barnason, S., Zimmerman, L., & Nieveen, J. (1995). The effects of music interventions on anxiety in the patient after coronary artery bypass grafting. *Heart & Lung, 24*(2), 124–132.

Blankfield, R. P., Zyzanski, S. J., Flocke, S. A., Alemango, S., & Scheurman, K. (1995). Taped therapeutic suggestions and taped music as adjuncts in the care of coronary-artery-bypass patients. *American Journal of Clinical Hypnosis, 37*(3), 32–42.

Byers, J. F., & Smyth, K. A. (1997). Effect of a music intervention on noise annoyance, heart rate, and blood pressure in cardiac surgery patients. *American Journal of Critical Care, 6*(3), 183–191.

Crago, B. (1980). *Reducing the stress of hospitalization for open heart surgery*. Unpublished doctoral dissertation, University of Massachusetts, Amherst.

Good, M. (1995). A comparison of the effects of jaw relaxation and music on postoperative pain. *Nursing Research, 44*(1), 52–57.

Good, M., Stanton-Hicks, M., Grass, J. A., Anderson, G. C, Lai, H., Roykulcharoen, V., & Adler, P. A. (2001). Relaxation and music reduce postsurgical pain. *Journal of Advanced Nursing, 33*(2), 208–215.

Heitz, L., Symreng, T., & Scamman, F. (1992). Effect of music therapy in the postanesthesia care unit: A nursing intervention. *Journal of Post Anesthesia Nursing, 7*(1), 22–31.

Locsin, R. (1981). The effect of music on the pain of selected post-operative patients. *Journal of Advanced Nursing, 6*, 19–25.

Mullooly, V. M., Levin, R. F., & Feldman, H. R. (1988). Music for postoperative pain and anxiety. *The Journal of the New York State Nurses Association, 19*(2), 4–7.

Nilsson, U., Rawal, N., Enqvist, B., & Unosson, M. (2003). Analgesia following music and therapeutic suggestions in the PACU in ambulatory surgery; a randomized controlled trial. *Acta Anaesthesia Scandinavica, 47*(3), 278–283.

Shertzer, K. E., & Keck, J. F. (2001). Music and the PACU environment. *Journal of PeriAnesthesia Nursing, 16*(2), 90–102.

Taylor, L. K., Kuttler, K. L., Parks, T. A., & Milton, D. (1998). The effect of music in the postanesthesia care unit on pain levels in women who have had abdominal hysterectomies. *Journal of PeriAnesthesia Nursing, 13*(2), 88–94.

Zimmerman, L., Nieveen, J., Barnason, S., & Schmaderer, M. (1996). The effects of music interventions on postoperative pain and sleep in coronary artery bypass graft (CABG) patients. *Scholarly Inquiry for Nursing Practice: An International Journal, 10*(2), 153–174.

Contributors

ര

DARCY DELOACH WALWORTH, MM, MT-BC, coordinated the music therapy program at Tallahassee Memorial HealthCare from July 2001–July 2003. During this time she implemented music therapy as procedural support for pediatric patients undergoing noninvasive procedures. She completed both her Bachelor and Master of Music Therapy degrees at The Florida State University.

CORENE HURT-THAUT, MM, MT-BC, is a therapist, educator, and researcher in neurologic music therapy with a Bachelor's degree in music from Western Michigan University and a Master's degree from Colorado State University. She has extensive clinical experience in neurologic rehabilitation, working at Wesley Woods Geriatric Hospital and the Center for Rehabilitation Medicine at Emory University for 3 years, and at Poudre Valley Hospital for 3 years, working with populations such as traumatic brain injury, cerebral palsy, autism, stroke, Parkinson's Disease, multiple sclerosis, speech and language disorders, and Alzheimer's disease. She is currently the coordinator for the International Neurologic Music Therapy Training Institutes and Advanced Fellowship Training at the Robert F. Unkefer Academy of Neurologic Music Therapy. She is on the teaching faculty of the Academy and in the Department of Music at Colorado State University. She has also been a Research Associate at the Center for Biomedical Research in Music (CBRM) for 8 years, participating in international and national research collaborations. At CBRM she started a research mentoring program for undergraduate music therapy students and a neurologic music therapy community outreach program for post-stroke patients in the community.

JENNIFER JARRED, MM, MT-BC, is currently employed as a supervising music therapist at Tallahassee Memorial HealthCare, Inc., in Tallahassee, Florida. There she provides music therapy services to pediatric patients in the Newborn Intensive and Intermediate Care Units, Pediatric Intensive Care Unit, preoperative waiting area, pediatric inpatient floor, procedural support, and Pediatric Rehabilitation. She received a Bachelor of Music Education at Louisiana State University and a Master of Music Therapy at The Florida State University.

SARAH JOHNSON, MM, MT-BC, created and developed the music therapy program at Poudre Valley Hospital in Fort Collins, Colorado. Over the past 15 years she has collaborated extensively with occupational, physical, and speech therapists at the hospital, working with neurologically impaired adults of all ages and children in the outpatient clinic developing and utilizing Neurologic Music Therapy (NMT) techniques. She has given numerous presentations at state, regional, and national conferences. Ms. Johnson is also an adjunct faculty of the Colorado State University Music Therapy Department, as well as an associate at the Center for Biomedical Research in Music. She received her Bachelor's degree in music therapy from the University of Minnesota and her Master's degree from Colorado State University.

Christine Tuden Neugebauer, MS, MT-BC, has been the music therapist in the Child Life Department at Shriners Burns Hospital in Galveston, Texas since 1994. She is the Music Therapy Clinical Training Director at SBH-G and currently serves on the American Music Therapy Association Internship Approval Committee. She serves as special project consultant with the Department of Pediatrics at the University of Texas Medical Branch in Galveston. She has lectured on music therapy and the treatment of pediatric burn injury at numerous conferences, hospitals, and universities throughout the country and abroad. She holds a Master's degree in counseling from the University of Houston–Clear Lake.

Volker Neugebauer, MD, PhD, is a physician-scientist trained in neurology, neurophysiology, and pharmacology. He presently holds the position of Associate Professor in the Department of Anatomy and Neurosciences at the University of Texas Medical Branch in Galveston, Texas. He is also Associate Member of the Graduate School of Biomedical Sciences. His research program combines behavioral, *in vivo* and *in vitro* electrophysiological, pharmacological, and biochemical techniques to analyze the role of the amygdala in the emotional-affective component of pain. He is the author of numerous original research articles and book chapters. His work is funded by grants from NIH/NINDS and John Sealy Memorial Endowment Fund for Biomedical Research.

Sheri L. Robb, PhD, MT-BC, is an assistant professor of music therapy at the University of Missouri–Kansas City. Robb earned her Bachelor of Music in music therapy at The Florida State University, Master's degree in early childhood special education at Auburn University, and Doctor of Philosophy in music education/music therapy at The University of Kansas. Dr. Robb serves as president of the Midwest Region of the American Music Therapy Association (AMTA) and serves on the Editorial Board of *Music Therapy Perspectives.* She presents regularly at local, regional, and national conferences. Dr. Robb's clinical research and professional publications focus on music therapy interventions for hospitalized children, specifically the use of music to promote coping behaviors in chronically ill children/adolescents.

Beverly J. Shirk, RN, BSN, CCRN, is employed as the Pediatric Trauma Case Manger at the Penn State Children's Hospital at Milton S. Hershey Medical Center in Hershey, Pennsylvania. She has previous experience as a staff nurse in the Pediatric Intensive Care Unit and as Clinical Head Nurse/Nursing Manager in the Pediatric Intensive/Intermediate Care Units at this facility. In the current role, she is responsible to oversee the acute care of traumatically injured children/families from admission through discharge. This includes coordinating the medical services, therapies, family education, and discharge planning along with the multidisciplinary team.

JAYNE M. STANDLEY, PhD, MT-BC, is the Ella Scoble Opperman Professor of Music at Florida State University. She is an active researcher and has published extensively in music in learning and music in medical settings. Most recently, she has specialized in research studies investigating the use of music with premature infants in the Neonatal Intensive Care Unit. Standley is a recipient of numerous awards and honors including the Publication and Merit Awards from the National Association for Music Therapy, a Florida State University President's Award for Teaching Excellence, and an FSU Award for Professorial Excellence. She is currently Editor of the *Journal of Music Therapy.*

JANICE W. STOUFFER, MT-BC, serves as the music therapist at the Penn State Milton S. Hershey Medical Center in Hershey, PA. Currently under the Department of Orthopedics and Rehabilitation, her primary clinical work involves children in the medical and rehabilitation hospitals. Research activity is focused on applications of music therapy with pediatrics in the critical care and oncology settings. Other clinical work includes adults in the hematology/ oncology and palliative care settings. Ms. Stouffer also serves as an adjunct faculty member of Elizabethtown College, Elizabethtown, Pennsylvania, supervising music therapy clinical practicum students.

MASAYO WATANABE, MD, is a physician at The Children's Mercy Hospital in Kansas City, who cares for kids with blood disorders and cancer. He grew up due to the efforts of a strict and musically talented teacher whom he called mother. He learned to play only three instruments, much to his mother's dismay and his family's amusement. Receiving education in Indianapolis, Boston, Kansas City, Japan, and North Carolina, he has many people to thank. Although Dr. Watanabe has a great love and respect for music, he has an even greater love and respect for children.

JENNIFER WHIPPLE, MM, MT-BC, has worked as a music educator and as a music therapist in psychiatric, crisis intervention, and medical settings. She currently serves as Chair of the Certification Board for Music Therapists Exam and Practice Analysis Committees, Southeastern Region Representative to the American Music Therapy Association Affiliate Relations Committee, and a member of the *Music Therapy Perspectives* Editorial Board. Ms. Whipple is a doctoral candidate in music therapy at the Florida State University. Her research emphases are infant and child development and communication disorders.